I Forgot That I Remembered

A collection of observations and experiences living with
Parkinson's disease, at times cleverly disguised as humor.

By Kevin T. Boekhoff

I Forgot That I Remembered

First Printing: November 2011

Second Printing: May 2012

Third Printing: December 2012

ISBN-13: 978-1481813426

Cover design by Katie Boekhoff

Photo by Katie Boekhoff

All scripture quotations in this book are taken from the King James Version (1611) of the Bible.

Acknowledgements

First of all I must thank my wife, Katie, for living Parkinson's disease with me, as well as helping me with clarity in my writing.

I also, thank my Lord Jesus Christ for helping with the spiritual aspect of life. I don't know why He allowed Parkinson's disease into my life, but He has shown me that this book is one of the purposes of it.

A special thanks goes out to Shantelle Boekhoff, Donna Cross, Joyce Heiser, and Mary Freeman for their proofreading efforts and encouragement.

I must not forget Susan Schrader, the editor of the National Parkinson Foundation South Dakota chapter newsletter, who felt my essays worthy of inclusion in the newsletter, and encouraged me to put together this book.

I also want to acknowledge the NPF/SD Newsletter, in which various forms of this book's pieces first appeared: "I Forgot That I Remembered," "Thoughts on Thoughts," "Yawnimals," "I Don't Smell So Good," Writing on Writing," "The Problem That Never Was."

2 Corinthians 1:2-6 Grace be to you and peace from God our Father, and from the Lord Jesus Christ. Blessed be God, even the Father of our Lord Jesus Christ, the Father of mercies, and the God of all comfort; Who comforteth us in all our tribulation, that we may be able to comfort them which are in any trouble, by the comfort wherewith we ourselves are comforted of God. For as the sufferings of Christ abound in us, so our consolation also aboundeth by Christ. And whether we be afflicted, it is for your consolation and salvation, which is effectual in the enduring of the same sufferings which we also suffer: or whether we be comforted, it is for your consolation and salvation.

Table of Contents

Introduction

Theories abound as to why Parkinson's disease affects some people and not others and how it manifests itself differently. Since other much more qualified authors have delved into that arena, I will only share my experiences, thoughts and reflections. You will find some to be humorous, some helpful, and some a little odd – like me!

I wrote this book to help me find humor in life, to encourage other "Parkies," to help those who know someone with Parkinson's disease, and to be a spiritual encouragement as well. My desire is to offer inspiration and hope to those with a chronic debilitating illness.

I am told that I have a skewed perspective on stuff. All I know is that I enjoy finding humor in things. All in all, I enjoy life. This book is just me finding humor in my struggles. I am a Christian so that element is interspersed within these pages, as well. Humor and the Lord's help are my greatest allies, so I included "My Uninvited Guest" to help anyone interested in knowing how Jesus can help and how they can know Him, too.

Over twenty-five years ago I discovered that I enjoyed creative writing when I read Patrick F. McManus and found I could write in a similar manner. Unbeknownst to him, he awakened the writer in me. In high school I attended the bonehead English classes that focused more on grammar than literature – praise God! Perhaps more of that stuck with me than I realized.

Writing is therapeutic – I have fun when I write,

consequently I feel better physically as well as emotionally. Then there is some inner need to inflict my humor on someone else – I hope you enjoy.

By the way, be sure to use the glossary for the definitions of the words I made up, and a couple others, as well.

If you would like more information on PD contact: National Parkinson Foundation South Dakota Chapter, 1000 N West Ave, Suite 220, Sioux Falls, SD 57104, 605-271-6113, www.npfsouthdakota.org. Email: info@parkinsonsd.org.

To reflect the unpredictability and haphazard traits of Parkinson's disease, I have left the essays in an unsystematic order, similar to the way they occur: plus, what works today many not work tomorrow, but then may work again the day after.

PMS

The other day we were in a second hand store, and the checker asked my wife, Katie, if I qualified for the senior discount. I had already come to terms with this aspect of my life when a waitress at a restaurant insisted I have their senior discount punch card even though I was not yet fifty-five[1]. At first I wondered why she thought I looked old, at least old enough to be considered a senior. However, I consented quietly, without protest, or enthusiasm, when I thought about having PD, which I felt qualified me for it, and I have since routinely taken advantage of it without any guilt. However, my wife, being of sound mind and honest demeanor said that I did not qualify for the discount at this store since my 55th birthday had not arrived, yet. I started for my wallet preparing to whip out my restaurant seniors' punch card as proof that I did, indeed, qualify. But Katie stood her ground. Even AARP considers me worthy of their benefits, but not Katie.

"You can have some of my years," proposed the guy behind us in line.

"Really?" I asked, "Do they come with experiences or are they basic models?"

"Whatever way you want them," he offered.

"Do you mean that you would give up your experiences? That's where you get your wisdom." I explained to him.

---

[1] I was not fifty-five at the time of this writing. I have turned fifty-five, yet still hold that it is too early to be a considered a senior citizen.

"Yup, you can have them whatever way you want them," he reiterated.

"Dear," I consulted my wife, "That is a great deal. What do you think? Should we take advantage of acquiring some "fully loaded" years?"

"No, it's not worth it. Someone else's experiences won't help you," she said, nixing my idea.

"But just think how smart I would be." I countered.

"You are assuming he is going to give you his good years; you could end up with the years he did stupid things, and thus, incur even more stupid tendencies." She reasoned.

She had me, I knew she was right. So, with my enthusiasm adequately squelched, I turned him down.

She did annoy me a bit, however, when she turned down the senior discount simply because I was underage. Who would have thought being underage would be a problem at fifty-four? At any rate, I believe that my PMS cancels out any such technicality. Oh yeah, PMS stands for Pre Maturely "Seniorized" - in other words, early onset old age. Essentially, PD ages one prematurely, so, I reason, the senior discounts should apply even if one is technically underage.

Next time, if confronted with being carded at fifty-four years old, I am going to claim I have PMS.

Writing on Writing

Recently, the editor for the NPF/SD newsletter, asked me to write on writing, I let the idea simmer in my mind a few days. Then, suddenly the urge to write prompted me to go to my computer. I sat down on my chair made from an automotive bucket seat, and looked around at my eclectically decorated desk. Die cast cars contrasted by Bev Doolittle calendar pictures surrounded me. I brought up a blank screen on my computer and began unloading the thoughts that had been ricocheting around my grey matter. I wrote for an hour or two - until my PD rendered my mind too foggy to compose anything. Then I ended up staring at the words on the screen and had to return to the project later.

During the night, I scribbled down some thoughts as they haphazardly stopped by to visit my consciousness. The following are some of these thoughts:

I have enjoyed writing for years, but it took PD to take away other distractions before I began writing creatively in earnest. Earlier in life, I would work on things with my hands, but PD makes my hands hurt if I do much with tools. My kids required family time. Various ministries needed my attention, and work demanded time. Writing creatively fell by the wayside – too much to do! Then PD came along and changed everything. Thus, the very thing I struggle with every single day; is the same thing that enables me to write – "parodoxicity" methinks.

I love the similarities and subtle differences in words, such as which write is the rite right? I enjoy word parts and rearranging them to create new words, as well as rearranging words to say the same thing in different ways. I rephrase and retell portions of the story until I enjoy them. Going over and over a story, editing it, polishing it, smoothing it, and getting the story to flow until it feels right is play. And, I can "play" at writing for hours at a time – unless my PD says, "Enough."

At times, spontaneous conversations can be difficult because the words do some serious evasive maneuvering at the most inopportune times. Writing, though, is a no pressure activity. My computer, complete with dictionary and thesaurus, lets me write, rewrite and write it over again, until I am satisfied with the wording. Through this process, my "voice" comes through. I have traded spontaneous wit for creative compositions.

Something that annoys me at times is that I must exercise my body in order to feel well enough to write. I dislike immensely the idea of taking time out of my day for physical activity. Actually, I hate exercise. I have things I want to do, things I need to do, and things I would rather do. But, I have found something I enjoy doing, which motivates me, to motivate myself to physical exertion.

This concept is similar to my need for spiritual exercise, such as reading the Bible, praying and attending church in order to keep my mind and attitude tuned up. I have found that focusing on something I like to do, keeps my mind off of the barrage of "cures" and "healings" touted freely by well meaning people, and thus, free from disappointment. Acceptance and trusting in God's grace frees me to enjoy life again. It lessens the distraction and frustration of finding a cure, or not, and also prevents me from falling for conmen of all kinds.

I find encouragement in doing something that I enjoy. I let it motivate me to do the necessary things like physical exercise. Both physical and spiritual discipline have their rewards – they help me do the things I want to do.

When I struggle with discouragement over having Parkinson's I read Philippians 1:6 "Being confident of this very thing, that he which hath begun a good work in you will perform it until the day of Jesus Christ," as well as a sign on my study wall that says: "It's not what happens to us in our lives that makes us into writers, it's what we make out of what happens to us."

I Am NOT Doing MS

"I am NOT doing MS (multiple sclerosis)." I emphatically proclaimed one day while "hobby-shopping" in my garage, "I am only forty-four years old and have too much to do to be sick."

I have loved cars all my life as attested to by my mother. She insists that I knew all the cars on the road by the time I turned five years old. My father, not a car lover, passed away during my seventh year, and mother remarried a couple years later. My step-father loved cars as well, so we experienced drag races and car shows together as I grew up. I ate, drank and breathed cars, so it seemed natural to go into a vocation working with cars – auto body repair. The idea of contributing to cleaning up the environment by taking a rolling eyesore and turning it into a compliment gathering eye-catcher appealed greatly to me. So, after high school I attended the a vocational school to learn the trade.

Some men love golf, or hunting and fishing, or carving or whatever. My favorite pastime consisted of sanding, working Bondo, sanding, priming, sanding, and spray painting cars. While "hobby shopping" on a 1974 Chevy pickup in 2001, soreness and stiffness began to hinder my progress, as well as my attitude. This went on day after day, until I got to the point that I even took my temperature a few times, but never had a fever. I saw the local MD. He said I just needed a massage. A massage! Since one of our church members had MS, and I had seen her struggles with pain, I began thinking it could be MS. I had seen several doctors through the years, but they sloughed it off as stress, depression, psychosomatic illness or, the one I really loved, that it needed to get more prevalent! More prevalent? Good night, it was prevalent enough, thank you very much.

I remember similar symptoms that occurred shortly after we moved to Montana about twenty-five years earlier. I had found a job at a small body shop. The building was comprised of many additions tacked on to one another and had been converted into a body shop with only a squirrel-cage fan for ventilation. Any flies, yellow jackets or other bugs that wandered into the building died shortly after. I didn't get to know the owner well because he died of cancer shortly after I started work there. The painter, Bruce, would joke about "our poor health" as he attempted to stop frequent nosebleeds. As with all the employees, he refused to wear masks of any kind because of the shop motto that "real men don't wear that sissy stuff." The owner's son showed me lumps under his skin but refused to go to the doctor. After a few months, I started to get very stiff and sore, and fatigue plagued my daily life. I thought of how lethargic the bugs got before they died. Since I could not get an answer from any doctors, I quit that job and began working as a janitor in the local hospital. After a year or so, the symptoms subsided and I felt fine.

Years later, when we founded a Baptist church in 1996, our income began to wane. I figured I could make better money repainting cars in the garage than working part time at a store, besides the convenience couldn't be matched. If I had an extra hour or two, I could "hobby-shop" a little bit. And, between buying project cars and repainting friends' vehicles, I kept fairly busy. But that is also when my symptoms came back to stay.

During my pastoral years, we went to many different doctors including the MS center in Denver. We left there knowing that the doctor felt something neurological was going on, but that it wasn't MS. He advised that we monitor the symptoms as they became more prevalent. It wasn't until we closed the church in 2006 and moved to South Dakota that we secured insurance through my job and pursued a diagnosis. Still, we waited through a year of the pre-existing condition clause before we could seek an answer. I found an internist that I liked and continued with him. Although he never said so to me, his notes stated that he suspected my symptoms were "somatoform" (my imagination), but he sent me to a neurologist anyway. The neurologist said that he felt something neurological was definitely going on. In his notes he said he suspected something in the basal ganglia. Finally, someone who agrees! But he wanted things to become more prevalent. Then, I went to the Mayo clinic, went through every test they could think of, and came back with no answer. An answer, even bad, was all we wanted.

A couple of months later a tremor started in my right hand. I called the local neurologist and he decided to try a low dose of Mirapex as a test to see if it changed anything. He said it was used to treat Parkinson's disease and that if nothing happened it wasn't PD, but if it helped, it would confirm Parkinson's. I discovered that, like clockwork, two hours after taking the med, my symptoms went away! My mind would clear and my muscles would relax. I felt I needed a good stretch when it kicked in. Thus, came the diagnosis. It wasn't psychosomatic! It wasn't my imagination! I didn't just need a massage! I wasn't a hypochondriac! I had an answer! I had credibility! The good news was that I had Parkinson's disease; the bad news was that I had Parkinson's disease.

I received my diagnosis with as much fanfare as a doctor would inform his patient that he had bronchitis. I didn't know what to expect other than I needed to take the medication, which I had no qualms about – it helped! I had researched MS (multiple sclerosis) prior to this, but knew nothing about PD (Parkinson's disease). So, I looked on the Internet, went to YouTube and other places and discovered that the future could really stink. I found out that PD did not go away, although the rate of progression varied with the individual. I didn't want to do MS, but the PD ride didn't look much better, just different.

After all this, I began thinking the warnings on the auto body product labels that said nerve or brain damage could result, are actually true. I discovered information on the Internet that autoimmune diseases such as MS and other maladies such as brain cancer, Alzheimer's and Parkinson's have been attributed to automotive paint. Since no one can point to anything specific that causes Parkinson's, and since PD has sprung up in the industrial age, it certainly could be the cause, and so I find nothing wrong with attributing my Parkinson's to that.

It turned out that I was correct, something was wrong and that I did not have to do MS. I get to do the Parkinson's disease journey.

It's Condensation not Perspiration

I have found in recent years that I am a good sweater, possibly due to PD. I can out-sweat the younger guys with no problem. It can be a relatively cool day, but throw in a little work and I will perspire. When people comment on how much I sweat, I tell them that it is not perspiration, it is condensation. My theory is that it is not that I am hot. On the contrary, it just may be possible that I am sooooo cool that condensation forms on me the same way it does on a cold can of pop.

My neurologist sent me to the Mayo Clinic in an attempt to diagnose what had demonstrated itself to be neurological problems. I experienced a myriad of tests, including one that required a collection of urine for 24 hours and then carrying the jug through throngs of people to a public drop off point. But the most memorable and tortuous one was the Easy Bake Oven test. The idea was to determine the extent of peripheral neuropathy. Lack of sweat means areas of nerve dysfunction. Therefore, lots of sweat means lots of nerve, right?

They wanted to see how much I could sweat and exactly where said sweat was emitted. So they covered me with a gold powder until I looked like Data on Star Trek. I then climbed on a gurney, and they rolled me into the "torture chamber". They allowed me to listen to my own CD as they turned on the contraption. I watched as the electric burners turned red and as they cycled on and off, black to red, hot to, well, hotter. I realized that I could now relate to how a turkey in a rotisserie felt, but after thinking about it, I concluded the turkey was dead and couldn't know how I felt! I was being cooked alive. So, my theory of "relativity" was experiencing distortion. I imagined my brain cooking. Would it be soft-boiled or hard-boiled by the time this was over? Did anyone remember to set the timer? Where is everyone? Did they go on break? Did they ever forget a roast in their oven at home? Hey, don't forget about me! When they come rushing back from break they'll remove my charred remains and blame each other for negligence.

I hate heat. As this incinerator did its job, I wondered, "Why would anyone want to lie on a beach in the hot sun like a turtle?" "Why would they subject themselves to such punishment?" I spent an entire hour, sixty minutes, 3600 seconds at 110 degrees basting in my own juices. Argh.

Occasionally, a nurse would have the audacity to ask how I was doing. As politely as I could muster, I would reply, "Awful." On one occasion I told her I understood a little bit of what hell is like. She laughed, or was it a chortle? She would return occasionally to reassure me that it wouldn't be much longer. I concentrated on my new music CD in a gallant effort to distract myself from the incessant, relentless scorcher. Based on the fact that most CD's contain forty-five minutes of music, I listened in misery to each song with the idea in mind that when the CD ended it wouldn't be long and I could escape this giant GE broiler oven. But this forty-five minute CD lasted for a time-span just short of eternity.

Finally, they let me out! The cool air felt wonderful as it evaporated the wetness covering me. Unbeknownst to me, that classy gold powder had turned purple when it reacted with the moisture emitted by my body. They held up a mirror – what an ugly eggplant! The purple people eater would have gone nuts if he saw me. They took me to a shower to wash off while they measured how much I had sweated. She said I was a good sweater – I already knew that. I didn't need to be broiled to tell her that! I don't remember the official amount, but I'm sure it had to have been close to filling a five-gallon bucket, an emesis basin and at least six bath towels! Along with the sweat, those containers held my cognition, energy and stamina – sweating sure takes a lot out of a guy. Besides the purple stuff didn't wash off easily, so I maintained a reddish purple glow for a couple of days.

But remember, it really wasn't perspiration, it was condensation. I kept my cool through it all.

A Memorable Day

Memorial Day weekend, 2010, I set my sights on doing something I have loved all my adult life. Most guys love fishing, golfing, hunting, flying model airplanes, ballooning, biking, or you fill in the blank. I love bodywork. I love fixing up and repainting cars.

I had been looking forward to doing some paintwork on my '92 GMC Sonoma. But that Saturday was filled with circumstances that hindered my plans and Sunday was the Lord's Day, so I was focused on that instead. Then Monday morning came! I got out my tools to remove the mud flaps and rear wheel-opening moldings.

I had dealt with stiffness and soreness in my hands for the past couple of years, but just using a screwdriver or ratchet hurt my hands much more than usual. Because of this I have trouble gripping things, which means I drop things a lot, yet still denied the problem. Even though I had allowed a body shop to fix my Sonoma after a lady sped through a blind intersection and I hit her Subaru Outback (pun intended). I wanted so badly to collect the insurance money and fix it myself. But my PD said, "No, just let a shop fix it...."

"This time." I countered, but only because it was winter and the truck would be down too long if I did it myself, besides her insurance was paying for it.

Back to my memorable day, I decided to mix a small amount Bondo to fix a little honey-do project. Just the stirring of the stiff putty-like substance caused the palm of my mixing hand to burn like fire.

So, that Monday, the reality of another appalling adjustment in my life hit home, the PD had stolen my favorite hobby. I grudgingly put away my grinder, sander and other tools, resigning myself to the fact that I couldn't do it. As I struggled with my emotions, my wife happened along, hugged me and encouraged me.

Later, I walked to the house and got cleaned up because I had learned something important that day. I figured out that I would have done like I had for years. I would have thoroughly enjoyed grinding, sanding, priming, and painting on my pickup all day and neglected something better.

Monday, I walked away **from something** I love - **to someone** I love. I spent the rest of the day in a leisurely manner with my wife. PD had forced me to slow down, yet helped me focus on something / someone more important. We spent time together talking and sharing like we did 30+ years ago. PD has changed my life, and at least regarding this point, for the better.

Thirty-one years ago on this weekend I married my wife, that Monday my marriage was realigned. Instead of spending our anniversary weekend painting a vehicle (which I have done in the past) PD made me re-evaluate what is truly important.

The Bible says *"Proverbs 18:22 Whoso findeth a wife findeth a good thing, and obtaineth favour of the LORD"*. It doesn't say finding a truck is a good thing, in fact in the long run, my wife, the help meet for me is infinitely more important than my hobby.

I Don't Smell So Good

I don't smell so good anymore. Nobody has had to inform me of this development; I have figured it out all by myself. It's not that I smell any worse, at least I don't think so, although I might not be able to tell. I may not smell so good to others, but then I haven't witnessed anyone with clothespins clamped on their noses. You see, my "sniffer's" olfactory cells work, but the receiver of said impulses doesn't work so well. This can be a blessing when there are things or people that smell like stink nearby, tainting the air. However, it is disappointing to be deprived of the pleasant aromas of hazelnut coffee, chocolate chip cookies and that new car smell.

My "schnozola" still works, but it isn't much of an appetite enhancer. I must press my smeller close to the odor emitter to be able to detect whether it is emanating a stench or a sweet smelling savor. Sometimes it lies to me and tells me of odoriferous things that are not there. On these occasions, I smell one of two things, the fragrance of lilacs in or out of season or the acrid pungency of barf. I much prefer lilacs. Most of the time I smell neutrality, which is really ok. There is nothing wrong with nothing. So I have decided that I will not be entering my proboscis in a "whifferama" in the near future because the fact remains that I don't smell so good.

Thoughts on thoughts.

During "off" times (times when the Parkinson's medication is not working) finding a thought is rather like shuffling through the lifeless desert terrain filled with skeletons of once viable thoughts. I turn over rocks and deadwood in hopes of finding some kind of life, any kind of life. I eventually discover a dried out, barely living idea, so dehydrated that it is barely recognizable as a full and flourishing concept once meditated upon. I nudge it with my toe in an attempt to see if there is any life in the thought, but I just bump it about with little puffs of dust that waft away and settle down in the sand. It has potential, but I can't get anything to happen no matter how long I work to revive it. Languishing lucidity – arghness to the max!

However, after the Levadopa kicks in, I have thoughts flying in my face vying for my attention. I capture one. It grows with my attention and nourishment. It embellishes itself with budding offspring – thoughts related to the thought, and those thoughts produce other related thoughts sometimes faster than I can record. Eventually a sermon or story has been created. If I let the thoughts come at random and entertain them briefly, "ridiculocity" results with highlights of nonsense and humorous episodes. Unlimited lucidity – what a concept!

I Hurt, Therefore I Am

I have found that with PD I am a champion "napper". I practice every day. My bed beckons me to spend quality time with it on a regular basis. It actually has become a wonderful friend. As I lie down, my pillow gets me in a head lock and my blankets, which are in league with my pillow, wrap around my body like a boa to keep me from escaping; but then, why would I want to break out of my cocoon when I am stiff and sore?

Fatigue is one thing but soreness/stiffness is quite another, yet they "cahooterize" a lot. When they attack, I hide under my covers and lie as still as I can until they go into hibernation. All is well as long as I don't move.

Every fall since 2001, as the weather turns colder, I experience more soreness and get rather grouchy for a day or two. Then it becomes so commonplace that it is rather like an annoying friend that hangs around in a persistent and perpetual manner. Finally, spring arrives and one day something changes. After thinking on the matter a bit, I deduce that the soreness/stiffness has disappeared. Yes! I am free! It is gone, never to return! I am all better! Yes! Yes! Yes! But within a day or two it returns and I feel like I am doomed to hurt forever. The good news is that summer turns into more good days than bad. Until it starts turning colder, and the cycle begins all over again.

As the years pass by, this phenomenon has progressively become more insistent, rendering me frequently under my covers in an unconscious state. Once I received my diagnosis, the consequent meds have given me ammo with which to fight back. Sometimes I can take a little extra Sinemet and win a round or two with an occasional extra allotment of energy and other times the meds do nothing and I am knocked out flat on my mattress.

Sometimes a sadistic synapse inside my head unleashes a surprise attack. I can be lying oh so contentedly under my covers when a myoclonic jerk (MJ) comes along. This causes a tsunami of muscle movement releasing a cacophony of screeching pain sensations which shatter my nap. MJ can come along at any time, but this is most aggravating because I must start the stillness process all over again. I hate waking up with a jerk!

Other times the pain isn't bad but the constant activity of twitching and dancing muscles intercepts the coming shipment of sleep. I think, "If only a cupful of sleep could make it through, but again, a case or two would be better."

Sometimes I wake up and ask Katie if someone threw a blanket party last night with me as the guest of honor. She denies any such activity occurred, but I feel like the recipient of a good beating anyway. I get up, take my Mirapex and Sinemet and return to bed and await the feeling that a good stretch would feel good. Prior to the medicinal benefits a stretch would just bring Charley Horse galloping over my body.

Before the meds I would spend my days pushing along through the stiffness/soreness and fatigue – a rather miserable existence at times. One day a coworker, who is not known for waxing eloquent, grew philosophical. He asked, "How do we know that this life is real. Maybe nothing is real at all. Maybe this is just all one big joke."

I replied, "I hurt therefore I am."

He informed me, "Well I hurt, too."

I said, "There ya go, reality hurts."

Aggravation Day

Parkinson's Disease has forced a role reversal between my wife and me and now I help with the domesticity in our home. One day when laundry day arrived, which is a bother of its own, I organized the clothes in piles of whites, colors and dark colors, then started to feed the clothing into the machines. Once the washer finished its agitation (a good word for it on this day), I stuffed wet clothes into the drier and turned the control knob, only to have it spin round and round without any cause or effect. Being reasonably intelligent, I surmised that something was amiss and pulled on the knob. It came off easily. I noticed that the plastic scabbard, AKA the "goes-on-ta", which was sticking off the back of the knob was cracked. This caused it to spin around on the "goes-in-ta", the shaft on the dryer; thus, no control.

"No problem, I'm having a good day. Besides I can fix this. All I have to do is push on the new one." I told myself, "I'll just hop in the Sonoma, run down to the local hardware store, buy a new one, replace it and do the laundry; thus achieving hero status on the home front."

Since the large national chain hardware store nearby carries appliances, I thought certainly they would carry parts. Not so. Though it went against everything masculine in me, I found someone with clerkish characteristics and asked him where I could find appliance control knobs.

"Just go down to aisle something-or-other and you'll find a whole rack of them."

He sent me to cabinet handles and knobs. I stood there

a moment, stunned. My Parkinsonian mind stripped a gear or two. Obviously, they wouldn't fit, would look stupid on a dryer, and would generate raised eyebrows on Katie's face. Plus I would subject myself to laughter, pointing and ridicule if another handyman type saw a cabinet knob on my dryer. I then found the clerk, who wasn't hiding, laughing or acting like he had pulled a prank, and patiently explained to him that they would not work and would look silly on a dryer. Then I asked him if they had just a simple universal pointy thing (perhaps using a different term than knob would help his understanding). I figured every hardware store should have universal appliance knobs that simply had a pointer in one spot of their circumference. Not so. The hassle potential was rising.

Since another hardware store was close by, I stopped in there. They said since they didn't carry appliances, they did not carry control dials for them, not even universal pointy knobs. This was getting annoying because they have a plethora of nuts, bolts, screws, washers and do-dads to fix things they do not carry.

Since I knew of an appliance parts warehouse, and since I still felt good, I dropped in there assured in the knowledge that even though I didn't like the counterman's attitude the last time I bought appliance knobs there, I could secure one. I showed the counterlady, countergirl, counteragent, counterperson, the count, or whatever she was, my broken part. She clearly didn't like being bothered with something as insignificant as a lowly control knob. After accessing the computer, making a call, and walking around in the back room awhile she said, "The factory discontinued making the part two months ago."

I asked, "Does your store have something else that would work? Like, a universal pointy knob?"

"No, we don't because they don't make universal pointer dials," she claimed. I restrained myself from asking who "they" were and why "they" would make such a decision without consulting some real people in the real world.

"Certainly, somebody must make universal appliance knobs. After all you can get many universal fit things in hardware stores." I replied.

"Nope. But, there is this appliance repair shop just up on the hill. Perhaps they could salvage something off of the old junk they have laying around," she said with a tone of disdain. Since I would not remember the directions, I asked if she could say them slowly so I could write them down. She complied, while making an inadequate attempt to hide her impatience. Some muttering took place as I walked to my truck, but subsided when I got out of earshot of the counter. When I climbed into the driver's seat, I found my frustration had grown to the point that he filled the entire passenger seat.

Since this apparent appliance salvage yard was located nearby, I took out the scrap of paper, tried to decipher the directions, but instead, embarked on some fruitless roving through the neighborhood near the prison. Up and down, round and round, with no results. I even consulted the knob in my possession to point the way by spinning it on the dashboard, but it didn't work. Why should it? It was broken!

We had purchased the appliances at a super-sized national chain hardware store, and even though my energy reserves were waning, I headed across town to check there. After all they should have it and I could go home. Nope, they did not have any. I expressed to the clerk my astonishment that they did not carry parts for their appliances - not even a universal pointy knob. He suggested that I get a zip tie to squeeze the cracked "goes-on-ta" tighter and put it back on. A zip tie? One of those plastic straps? Yup, that's what he meant. He took me to bags of them, even though I only needed one. How could one possibly get a zip tie tight enough to secure a knob on the "goes-on-ta"? Did this guy go to knucklehead school? Frustration turned into irritation, which took up more room in the cab of my small truck.

Since a competing chain hardware store was located across the freeway, I stopped in there. I could handle one more stop. Same story, except this guy vigorously implored me to call their super duper parts number because, "They would have it – they ALWAYS have what no one else does."

I called. Nope, the factory does not make that control knob anymore. I knew that! I simply needed my annoyance invigorated. Irritation joined frustration leaving little room for me in the cab of my pickup.

Since I had previously bought things from a little appliance repair shop located on my way home, I pulled into the parking lot only to find that it had gone out of business! The grump factor kept growing.

Since I noticed an appliance store further down the same street, I stopped in. I could handle one more stop, but not any more. I think I must have interrupted the salesman's nap, because of his "cantakerosity". I told him what I needed and without a word he turned and walked away. I wondered whether he was angry with me, returning to his nap or going to the parts section to check. I followed him. He went into the back room and found some small parts bins, pawed through them, shook his head and actually spoke! He suggested just putting a vice grip on the "goes-in-ta". A vice grip? How tacky does that look? My handyman ranking would be stripped from me and I would be ostracized by mechanically minded men everywhere. And, worse yet, I would open myself up to ridicule from my wife. No thanks. He seemed insulted that I wouldn't even consider his idea, turned his back on me without a word and returned to his pillow. Exasperation joined frustration and irritation. I elbowed them over as I squeezed into the driver's seat, enveloped in defeat and went home and rested.

I had not found any help, but my thinker had been stimulated. After my nap, a thought interrupted my pout. I decided to rummage through my stuff to find a radiator hose clamp small enough to squeeze the knob housing securely onto the shaft sticking out of the drier. I found one in my organizer filled with do-dads, whatchamacallits, and thingamajigs and in two minutes had it fixed! The "goes-on-ta" has stayed on the "goes-in-ta" wonderfully and nobody can see my "cobblized" improvisation.

But then I found myself grumping that this two minute repair job took three hours, a long recovery nap, and several gallons of gas when the solution resided in my garage all the time. It's curious that even success can be aggravating.

Bodily Betrayal

My body and I used to get along quite well. We had symbiotic relationship – a mutually dependent one. We usually worked in unison. I told it what to do and it did it. Sometimes I endured consequences for overdoing it. Other times I injured it. I never intentionally abused it, except for some instances when I was young and the "stupidaline" made me do it. (All men have a "stupidaline" gland, but it is overactive in young guys and causes them to do stupid things. Old men suffer from a "stupidaline" deficiency and thus, never have any fun).

Since PD, my body and I find ourselves at odds frequently. I want to do something, and it refuses. For example, I'll say, "I want to open this pop bottle." My body says, "Oh yeah? Not today buddy." At this point, my determination kicks in and I endure thirst until I can open it later, or delegate it to someone else. It takes great resolve to tough it out when my body betrays me, let me tell you.

Sometimes, when the order for words comes in to the vocabulary center of my brain, a gremlin substitutes another word and ships it out for delivery to the speech department. He doesn't necessarily use synonyms, either. Some people look at me strangely, and I try to analyze the replay of the tape of what I said in my mind, others will volunteer my malapropism to correct me, and others enjoy a good laugh. The frustration lies in the fact that I think I am saying what I want, but experience bodily betrayal instead.

Sometimes my body demands something to eat by

threatening a crash. If I don't eat something, the crash will, in fact, manifest itself in all its frustrating glory. On the other hand, sometimes eating helps and other times it does not. The conundrum is whether my body is lying or has slipped into intimidation mode. Regardless, the consequence seems to be that my body gains unnecessary flabbiness (as if there is necessary flabbiness, hmmm).

Just about everyday my body pulls a leg out from under me – or it tries to. Without my cane, and sometimes with it, I find myself meeting the ground unexpectedly and abruptly. The surface material encountered dictates whether I acquire marks or not. Nevertheless, it is not a pleasant experience. Bodily betrayal can be unpredictable.

Sometimes my body says I need to use the facilities, but then when I get there I discover it is a false alarm. Then later on it decides, at an extremely inconvenient time, to declare an emergency of an imminent sort. I find myself rather irritated with such scenarios and fuss at my body, "I could have gone three minutes ago when I was in the store, NOW you must go? NOW?" When this occurs my body laughs maniacally. Betrayed again!

When I need to sleep, my body betrays me by getting my days and nights mixed up. I am wide awake at 3:00 AM; then, when I need to be awake I experience a sleep attack. This is most troublesome when Katie asks me a question, and I fall asleep before I can answer. It seems to annoy her, somehow. My body can betray me in this same manner while driving, which is not a good thing because I should be alert and awake for such an activity. Therefore, I do not drive far;

in fact, I do not drive at all, unless I feel reasonably vigilant.

Which reminds me of crashes – the sudden onset of symptomatic behavior. I like feeling good, but I get sick and tired of feeling sick and tired. Generally, my body betrays me in this arena, by soreness, stiffness and fatigue. Sometimes, though, malaise (feeling just plain icky) grabs all the attention in this three ring circus called life. When I feel a crash coming on, I end up spending quality time with my pillow.

It seems the only thing consistent these days, due to PD, is inconsistency.

The "Yawnimals"

I have recently discovered the reason I yawn, go cross-eyed, nod repeatedly and snore publicly, especially late in the evenings. "Yawnimals." Yes, they do exist. They are difficult to spot due to their changeling characteristics which allows them to blend into their surroundings. They may look like common everyday items, but as soon as you are comfortable, they will scurry along the baseboards and dash from one shadow to another seeking to remain in obscurity as they stalk their prey. You have seen them, they are those glimpses that just seem to be a movement in the corner of your eye, but when you quickly look, nothing is there. "Yawnimals."

In my home, they hide behind my Lazy Boy and move as quietly as any puma in stealth mode. I have never sensed their approach in any way. They use a warm fuzzy strategy, feigning affection, which is very effective. I have no idea they have been at work making me feel oh so comfortable, when suddenly, I find myself yawning. Argh, the "yawnimals" are here! They are on the move and I am their quarry! I have more reading to do, but yawning leads to catnaps. I know more light and cold will send them scurrying back to wherever they live, but since that is not comfortable for me either, I usually end up dimming the lights, covering up with an afghan and settling in again – before long I yawn again. Those "yawnimals!"

Sometimes they congregate behind my Lazy Boy until they have formed a swarm. Then suddenly, yet just as stealthily as ever, they attack. This happens so subtly that I am rendered unconscious almost instantly and don't know of the attack until my book hits the floor losing my page. Plus, I must now, with great effort accompanied by grunts, groans and grumbling retrieve said book from the floor to find my place only to discover that I don't remember what I was reading. Those "yawnimals!"

I have also discovered that when I have taken my Mirapex the "yawnimals" go through a metamorphosis that makes them much more aggressive. They change from a warm fuzzy approach that softly and slowly brings on sleep to an all out frontal assault called a sleep attack. It can happen anywhere at anytime. They remind me of the warm cuddly gremlins, from the movie of that name, that turn into evil leathery things at night. Everything is fine, then suddenly I wake up to the distant laughter of those evil "yawnimals."

"Yawnimals" don't just live in my home, they ride along in my car, shop in the same stores I do and even hang out in the same cafes that I like. Personally, I believe they stow away in my pockets.

They also reside where people flock together. I have witnessed their work by watching the people during assemblies. For example, as a teacher instructs the students, I have noticed their attacks progressing through a crowd. It begins with an individual yawning and then progresses through the group causing congregational nodding of heads. Some people succumb easily and emit curious sounds, which disturb those nearby. Others produce unintentional verbalizations when they have been "snoozified," which embarrasses the victim, but has an entertainment factor to those close enough to hear.

A most disturbing occurrence would be sleep-walking especially in a people infested area! Just imagine waking up at a restaurant with a different group of people than you arrived with. Personally, my biggest fear is to be swarmed by "yawnimals" while preaching and fall asleep on the pulpit! Would the people wake me or just quietly leave, allowing me to wake up alone sometime later?

"Yawnimals" – they do exist and are a serious menace to my consciousness.

Stuck Foot

One Sunday I experienced another revolting development. I was headed to teach a class which required descending the steps into the church basement. Suddenly, I found myself descending them with various parts of my body in a noisy, accelerated fashion.

I started out with my briefcase and Bible in my right hand and a frappuccino in my left. I must have had another experience of sticky feet. (This occurs when one or both of my feet refuse to cooperate while the momentum of my body keeps the upper part moving. I have never been able to discern exactly what happens when this occurs as it happens in quite an unexpected and speedy manner). Evidently, a foot stuck. I remember stepping downward a few steps and suddenly the linoleum tile floor slapped me on my back hard enough to knock the wind out of me and thwacked the back of my head, as well. Meanwhile, frappuccino droplets showered down as my mug skittered across the Fellowship Hall and my briefcase and Bible skidded to a stop next to me.

I looked around hoping no one saw me experience my frappuccino shower. However, no one saw me, which prompted the thought that I could have been seriously injured and would have lain there in the midst of my personal belongings indefinitely. I didn't want anyone to have seen and yet wanted someone to have seen, argh, I am my own conundrum!

Since my wind had been knocked out, I found my second wind, gathered my wits and debris, and with each step my frappe-coated soles squeaked across the linoleum and ascended the aforementioned steps in retreat. Since the bongo drums in my head needed attention and a change of clothes was in order, I returned home. I am glad that no one had to see a disheveled, coffee stained, giant sized lint roller leaving the church in defeat.

However, by the end of the evening, the entire church knew about it and was praying for me! Therefore I was glad my wife had shared a prayer request for me and that they knew.

Lost in the "Bewilderness"

The thick darkness of this moonless night amplified the Christmas lights strewn across the shrubbery and house. Why were there Christmas lights in October? At least I think its October. What street is this? Where am I? I sat there by the side of the road, bewildered looking quite like a "bewildebeast" lost in the "bewilderness." I hate when my Parkinsonian brain does this.

One October evening after prison services, I unwillingly and unwittingly found myself engaged in an unplanned trip into the "bewilderness." Since I had been unable to participate in the prison ministry lately and because I had enjoyed a great day, one filled with lucidity and very little fatigue, I decided to attend that evening. At some indistinct point during the services I could feel my brain disengaging. When the preacher asked me an address for a Bible verse, my brain came up with something like, phzzzzt, but a Bible savvy inmate spoke up and saved me from public futility. After the services, during the fellowship time, attempts to contribute to conversations stressed me a bit. As far as I know, I made it without anyone suspecting my brain was malfunctioning.

I exited the prison, and crossed the road through the darkness that had invaded the area during the services and had turned the city into a "bewilderness." As I waited my turn to pull out from my parking space on the side of the road, a customized Harley motorcycle roared by with the framework emblazoned with blue neon lights, striking me as a demonized Smurf bike from hell and messing with my already befuddled gray matter.

After a moment, I started my Sonoma, pulled out and drove along the familiar road. The name didn't matter just as long as it took me home. At the light I turned right and dropped downward and eastward as the road curved to the right and intersected with a street, on which I turned left and meandered on until I reached Cliff Avenue. I vaguely recalled this was the correct route. I turned right and suddenly there were many kinds of lights, lanes, vehicles and more lights. Pressure to proceed at a hurried and harried pace forced my brain to make decisions quicker than it really wanted to. Praise God, traffic was light. The usual behavior of red lights gave me frequent reprieves. I traveled through each traffic light as though it were another hurdle cleared toward my goal - home. The twenty-five foot statue of Mr. Bendo at an automotive exhaust repair shop manned the main combination checkpoint/ landmark of a left turn I needed to make. I navigated into familiar territory, I'd be home soon, no problem.

Somewhere along 15th Street, or was it called 12th Street (I was unsure) I ended up on an unfamiliar side street. Houses and trees lined both sides of the street with darkness oozing out from the night, threatening to choke out my headlights. Suddenly the street started bending. How do streets bend? Oh, they don't, they curve. I pulled over. Which street curves? Where was I? What do I do? I called Katie, to talk me home, but no answer. (She had become separated from her cell phone, rendering her unreachable for the rest of the night). I decided to drive until I found something familiar and then I could get myself home. It never crossed my mind to turn around, retrace my tracks, and rediscover Mr. Bendo. I came across road construction signage. A red light gave me a respite from the pressure of a decision until I saw a car go through, guiding the way for me. I drove aimlessly for quite a while turning here or there, but all the neighborhoods looked the same – houses and trees swallowed up in blackness.

The numbness of my mind held the anxiety at bay as I wandered. I came across a house decorated with Christmas lights as if I were caught in an episode of the Twilight Zone. After driving awhile, suddenly a main thoroughfare appeared! I turned right. Traffic, lights, pressure, go, go, go, vehicles and more lights. In the midst of the chaos I found an oasis of hope, a lighthouse of familiarity – a fast food place specializing in roast beef sandwiches. Home was near! I proceeded along by a well-known grocery store and a farm supply store; yes indeed. I turned at the auto parts store and tooled contentedly in the knowledge that I would soon see the maple trees of home in my headlights. I turned at the stop sign into the darkness accentuated by houses and trees. What happened? Where am I? I drove until I saw the fast food place again! Whew! I turned, drove past an auto body repair shop, turned onto the busy street again, whatever it was called. A number I think, 12th, 10th , 15th or something like that. Anyway, I turned at the auto parts store and did the same thing two or three more times. What is wrong! I hate the "bewilderness!"

On one of my circuits I turned the opposite way at the fast food place and found myself at a familiar light on some street with a number for a name. I turned left on it. Then darkness obscured all familiarity again. I live on one of these streets, I know I do. I turned on one and it started bending. I hate it when streets bend as I travel on them – rather disorientating. I drove up and down streets until I noticed the two humongous maple trees illuminated by streetlights that indicated my yard! I drove in the driveway in a stupor. I was home, yet rejoicing just didn't come. I was home and just wanted to go to bed, ignore the bad dream like I usually do with nightmares and wake up in the morning without a memory of it.

The next day I discovered that the search was not over. I had put my things away, "away" being the key word. I had to ferret out various articles of clothing that I had worn that night. While on this pursuit I found my shirt on a hook in a different closet and my belt rolled up and put on my desk amongst office supplies.

Oh, the adventures of a "bewildebeast!" I am just glad PD generated bewilderment occurs only occasionally.

The "Fangster"

I do know the difference between right and wrong decisions. One brings accolades, awards and pats on the back, while the other brings shame, embarrassment and shunning from society. The problem comes in when I discover that I was right, when I thought I was wrong. Originally, then, was I wrong when I was right or was I right when I was wrong?

This philosophical dilemma occurred when an intruder of the creepy-crawly sort invaded my territory and commenced to biting my leg. This little "fangster" bit me nine times!

There I was, kicking back in my easy chair on a Thursday evening when I felt something odd. I said to no one in particular that if I didn't know better I would think some insect was biting me. My wife, the only other person in the room, showed little concern probably thinking I was just muttering to myself about some inconsequential thing again. However, it turned out, when I turned in for the night, that I discovered a series of nasty swollen red spots that begged to be scratched. I showed Katie the trail of bites up my calf and knee left by some unseen bug. I had been right! At the time, though, I had convinced myself that I was wrong. Had I believed that I was right and taken appropriate action, I would have been able to fend off the little fangster and, thereby, have prevented some bites. Thus, I was wrong in thinking I was wrong.

I closely inspected my trousers, but the culprit had

split. I looked around the room, but didn't see any multiple-legged malefactors. I deemed them spider bites. What else could it be? The weather had turned cold. Any outdoor bugs were moving in slow motion due to the fact that their bodily fluids were like sludge and hindering their movement. I was unable to experience satisfaction in disposing of the perpetrator. He was on the lam somewhere in my house.

The knowledge of a creeping thing on the loose in the close vicinity can bring feelings of little feet roaming around on my arms and legs. However, when I check it out, I find my imagination has been messing with me and that I am wrong.

Within a couple of days the spots had grown zit-like with whiteheads. Then, I began feeling lousy – foggy brain, stiff neck, body aches, joint pain in the left leg and a headache. I thought I had a fever, but was wrong – unless the thermometer lied when it said my temperature was ninety-two degrees. I could have been right about a fever, but I'll never know. Anyway, the symptoms were very similar to a bad PD day, so I decided that it was simply the Parkinson's running in overdrive for the next two days. It turns out that was wrong.

On Friday, I called my daughter to access the internet to see if I was right about spider bites. She did so and verified my theory. Her concern consisted of what kind of spider bit me. I really didn't care about his or her heritage. But in reality, the issue was venom strength and the consequences thereof. My thoughts turned to an occasional wolf spider that I had seen in the basement. I thought that perhaps one of those had bitten me, but decided I could be wrong.

Saturday, I called the ask-a-nurse about the bites. She seemed concerned about anaphylactic shock, hyper-allergic reactions to the venom and such like. I answered a list of questions and ended up with the advice not to scratch them, but monitor them, take an analgesic (Tylenol, Advil, Bufferin and the like), and if anything changes have a health professional look at them. I was already following her advice, so, I was right!

That evening, I turned on the light as I entered the bathroom and clinging to the wall was a large, black wolf spider. I least I think it was a wolf spider. I didn't ask him, I didn't take his picture, I didn't capture him for interrogation purposes - I grabbed a tissue and ended his life. You may take issue that I invoked capital punishment on a spider without due process of law. However, I may be wrong, but he looked evil. He looked guilty to me. Besides he had broken the creepy-crawly trespassing rules of this household and thus paid the ultimate price for his transgression. I feel I killed the correct spider because no other spiders have shown their fangs in my house since then.

Monday, I compared my bites with photos on the internet. They lined up with general spider bites - wolf spider bites fit into the category. I could not find a mug shot of the specific "fangster" that had shown up in my bathroom, but did discover one very similar out of the 250 kinds of wolf spiders. Thus, I deemed myself right again.

Originally, I thought something was biting me, but I

pooh-poohed the concept, which allowed the spider time to inflict more damage. I was right, but thought I was wrong, then discovered that I had been right after all. I was right when I suspected a spider bite caused my two days of being under the weather, but dismissed it as my Parkinson's. I was wrong to think I wasn't right.

The unanswered question still hangs in midair: was I wrong when I was right or was I right when I was wrong?

Going Forward in Full Reverse

Everything's "wackbards" these days. Oh, I'm still going forward, but Parkinson's disease has reversed many things, such as the transposition of our marital roles. Katie, has become the breadwinner and clears the snow or mows the lawn, depending on the season, while I am learning to carry out a few of the household duties. Some may call me a "Cinderfella," but I prefer to say that I am going forward although in full reverse.

For example, I never realized all the idiosyncrasies involved with washing clothes. Katie is attempting to train me to separate the laundry according to colors, textures and types of material; not dirtiest, kinda dirty and almost clean. She says to segregate the white stuff from all colored garments, because putting something red in with my white shirts would turn them into pink blouses. I learned one must put the correct product(s) in the wash or weird things can happen to shirts – recently, I ended up with strange spots on some rendering them unsuitable for public appearances. The soaps, boosters, and softeners we buy come with clever plastic measuring cups/lids so that I can gauge the exact combination needed for each unique grouping of contents; this goes contrary to my usual style of a "glub" or two of soap in the water and telling the machine to go.

That's another thing, you can't just tell it to "go". After selecting the water temperature, one must analyze things a bit. Do I want to put it on "presoak," "soak," "delicates," "colors," or "whites"? No problem with the colors and whites, but what is the difference between soak and presoak? Don't they both soak? Why soak the stuff before you soak the stuff? Does the agitator somehow agitate delicately? I learned that phrase is an oxymoron when I tried to delicately agitate Katie – bad idea.

Why all the different settings? Can't the machines just say "off" and "on"? Better yet, "stop" and "go"? I am still in training and may be until the day I die because I have to be retrained every week. Still things are moving forward, although in full reverse.

I even do some food prep – if it does not require hand held power tools, or should I say, appliances. One day, I needed to mix cookie dough. I figured the hand-held mixer was simply a drill with churning attachments. How hard could it be? I discovered that sticks of butter create butter-filled dough balls unless thoroughly thawed. Since my hands hurt gripping such things, I turned it on high to get the job done more quickly. However, the cleanup from that strategy cancelled out any time savings. Katie salvaged my cookies. I have changed my strategy. I now buy the homemade style bakery cookies at the grocery store. Katie felt the anxiety of reversing roles through the cookie caper as much as I did. Yet we are still going forward - in full reverse.

I even go to the grocery store occasionally – with the lifeline of my cell phone so I can contact her for advice or directions. Recently, the grocery store I frequent decided to rearrange things AND take down the signs with clues at the end of each aisle. Do they realize that this could cause severe stripping of the gears in a man? Since guys don't like asking for directions, men were wandering in a lost and forlorn manner throughout the store talking incoherently to themselves. One particular guy and I kept bumping into each other and fussing about this revolting development. I happened across a clerk and complained to him about this disorienting situation. He said he understood and asked what I was looking for. I related one item on my list. He escorted me to it and "poof" disappeared. I still had several items to go. I began fussing and talking quietly to myself. Even if I resorted to my lifeline, I couldn't call my wife for help because she wouldn't know either. They rearranged the entire store!

I put Ranch dressing on the list, and Katie had told me to buy only Hidden Valley. Well, that narrowed it down, no problem. However, I discovered a large area of several shelves devoted solely to the ten different varieties of Hidden Valley ranch dressing! Now came the dilemma; do I pick something out and hope I get it right, or use another lifeline? I used another lifeline. We needed the Original flavor, not fat free and not "light." I later found out that the same problem exists with facial tissue, toilet paper and paper towels. Praise God for cell phones and a patient wife.

Now when people ask me how I am doing, I can say I am going forward in full reverse

Get Up, Get Up, Let's Go

Katie tells me that I think differently than other people. For example, some people complain that they wake up in the night and can't sleep. Then when they do get to sleep they can't wake up after the alarm goes off. Well, this is how it works in my mind.

The other day at 3:42 AM I woke up and my body said, "Get up, get up, get up, get up, get up, get up; let's go-go-go-go-go-go-go-go!"

I said, "No way, it is 3:42 in the morning, we are going back to sleep."

My body replied, "But do you know how often I feel this good? We have been battling this Parkinson's thing for over nine years. We feel good now, so let's not waste it. Let's get up, get up, get up, get up, get up, get up; let's go-go-go-go-go-go-go!"

I refused to budge, "No, we are going back to sleep until the alarm goes off at 5:51, then we are going to snooze for nine minutes and then get up when that alarm goes off again."

My body sighed heavily and stared off into the blackness, pouting. Suddenly, the alarm went off with all-out obnoxious fury at 5:51. I did not notice the passing of time – unconsciousness does that.

"Is the alarm in cahoots with my body?" I wondered. I hit the snooze button and snoozed 'til 6:00, at which point my alarmist clock returned to making nasty noises.

My body said, "We're not getting up now."

I ask, "Why not?"

It argued, "Because you wanted to go back to sleep and so we are going to sleep."

I made my body get up anyway, and drug it about for a couple of hours before it finally woke up, yet not to the degree it was at 3:42 am.

All the while it reminded me, "You should have gotten up when I told you to and you wouldn't be fighting the fatigue now."

I replied, "Yeah, right. You have lied to me about fatigue before."

"But you could have gotten something done when I gave you the chance." I knew my body had me on this one.

Later in the day, I told my co-worker about this scenario and he looked at me incredulously, and said that he had NEVER had such a problem.

Perhaps Katie is right after all, maybe I don't think like other people.

This is something I wrote some time ago and as I was rereading and editing it, it reminded me that we should not be wasting our time *(Ephesians 5:16   Redeeming the time, because the days are evil)*. No one knows how much time they have but those with chronic illness know that their days of service to the Lord have been shortened. Taking advantage of lucid moments becomes more important. Maybe we can't do what we used to but we can do what we can when we can.

I Forgot That I Remembered

No ignition regarding my cognition occurred the other day – I forgot that I remembered.

I usually take preemptive steps to intercept times of memory issues. For example, every Tuesday I bring the devotional at my church's men's prayer breakfast. The night before I make sure I have the message tucked in my Bible on the text verse's page, thereby avoiding the problem of not remembering where said verse is in the Bible and not having to depend on the Table of Contents or even remembering that there is a Table of Contents on a bad day – especially in front of people. I then put my Bible in a conspicuous place so that its presence reminds me that it is to go with me. Each day is unpredictable, so I cannot plan tomorrow's events, just prepare for possible difficulties. But this is not a normal "Sometimers" occurrence, but a seriously disconcerting event.

However, this Tuesday, despite my strategy, I forgot that it was Tuesday. I ate breakfast at home and, despite my "Novacaine brain," went for my morning walk. When I got several blocks away, a serious no-nonsense rain began. As I trudged back home, and I had no more energy than a trudge, I came across a garbage man, one that I had had run-ins with on previous Tuesdays (he doesn't like pedestrians to "get in his way"); thus, I remembered that I had forgotten where I should be at that very moment – at the restaurant for men's breakfast! And I am the leader of said breakfast! So, I began to plod along at a faster pace toward home. Once there, I grabbed my Bible, forgetting my lunch and mug of Bengal

Spice Tea. I climbed into my 1992 Sonoma and headed out. I arrived a little early for work. While sitting there waiting for the business to open, I noticed my Bible on the other seat. Guess what? I had forgotten that I remembered the men's breakfast! Now it was impossible to get there before everyone else was gone. Argh!

I had forgotten what I should have remembered, remembered that I had forgotten, and then forgot that I remembered! I figured I better write this down before I forgot! Hey, I remembered!

The Headache with Migraine Meds

"Argh, how is a guy supposed to get into this thing," I fussed, and I am good at fussing. But this provided a bona fide reason to fuss!

I suffer from occasional migraine headaches for which my neurologist prescribed Maxalt. I dutifully purchased my prescription and brought it home. The stuff is only to be used if I feel a migraine coming on; consequently, I had to wait for the next event.

Sometimes my migraine would begin with an odd visual lightshow called an aura. One day sitting at my computer writing, a small "pow" sign appeared in the lower left corner of my vision (A "pow" sign is the shape that indicates a loud noise in cartooning). This little pulsating "pow" sign expanded in size until it filled my computer screen. Inside the pulsing "pow", sign everything was so distorted that I couldn't read. Once it expanded outside of my field of vision, an incredible headache started. The directions said to take the Maxalt as soon as I notice an aura, my problem on that occasion was that I didn't know what had happened.

Usually my headaches start in the night and the pain wakes me up. This is especially annoying because by then it is raging full-force. At that point, bright lights are painful, movement hurts, loud noises aggravate, and patience is not nearby.

It is in this condition that I wrestled with the pharmaceutical paper bag until I tore it open to free my prescription to stop my brain from hurting. Then I opened the Maxalt box and found a plastic box. I popped open the lid only to find foil packages, which refused my efforts. I had to turn on a light, endure the pain and attempt to focus on the tiny letters that won't stay still. There is a line at the top of that read, in tiny print, "fold" so, I folded it back and forth and then tried to tear it from the edge, then from the other edge. I looked at it again. I found there is a "notch" in the middle, not like the usual notched packages I dealt with on a daily basis. I tried to tear it and looked at it again. I realized that I was supposed to fold the foil envelope, and then tear at the notch. Nothing happened! Was I supposed to fold it in half again? Exasperated, I fumbled noisily through the junk drawer in the kitchen for a pair of scissors; which I used to cut it open. I found the pill, but it was still inside a bubble package! Argh. Since I had the scissors already, I cut it open without trying to read any how-to-open directions and put it under my tongue as per instructions. Guess what! It worked! Who "woulda thunk it" after all that?

My question is: why do they do this to someone with a migraine? Now throw in Parkinson's, too. Just opening all the packages to get to the headache medicine can cause a headache!

The "Contortium"

As I headed out for work one winter morning, the windshield fogged up on my '92 Sonoma despite the fact that I had the defroster on full speed. In fact, it made it worse! The sickeningly sweet smell of antifreeze tried to engage my not-quite-awake brain as I thought about the problem. At the next stoplight, I reached under my seat and pulled out a rag. I wiped off the slimy residue, confirming that the defroster was, in fact, misting antifreeze on the windshield. My mediocre diagnostic skills concluded that a leaking heater core was behind this revolting development.

Over the next few days, the problem worsened. One day I noticed the passenger side floor mat had a puddle of green fluid that surged forward like a miniature tsunami whenever I applied the brakes. Thoughts of praise and worship swirled inside my head. Not. I grumbled. I am sure I heard a ka-ching sound every time I blinked and the idea of contorting myself in the small cab of the Sonoma excited me as much as being force-fed a plate of kohlrabi. Since, my PD had begun taking its toll, I routinely returned from work exhausted. Therefore, I put off the inevitable until the next Saturday.

First thing the next Saturday morning, I felt statuesque - stiff and sore as a statue. I set out to enter the "contortium" anyway. I consulted a repair manual specifically for my pickup that I had acquired from a rummage sale some time in the not so recent past. That someone sold it cheap should have been my first clue, I suppose. I referenced the heating/cooling system, which told me to go to section three, page ten. However, page ten talked about air conditioning. I paged forward, nothing. I paged backward and found it on page nine. That should have been my second clue. However, I had found it and, thus, confidently, yet in an inflexible manner, embarked on removing the leaky heater core.

The book even had a diagram corresponding to the instructions. After disconnecting the battery and draining the coolant, it said to remove, what it called, the "modular duct" (a cover that connected to the ductwork), disconnect the hoses, then the mounting bolts – a quick and easy project. The book lied, or, should I say, omitted important information. The book failed to mention that the dashboard was in the way. Evidently they based the book on a vehicle with no dashboard in it. Weird. The repair manual also failed to include instructions on dashboard removal!

I entered the "contortium" by moving the passenger seat all the way back, squirming in, and lying on my back on the floor. I rolled on my left shoulder and twisted my head to look under the dash. My reward for making my body hurt more than it already did was a plastic shield not mentioned in the book. I could see nothing of any importance. I wriggled out and consulted the book again. Nope, the wording hadn't changed and the omissions hadn't magically appeared. Rats.

I began taking off various covers, plastic pieces and the glove box in an attempt to find access to the modular duct, but all I accomplished was scattering pieces everywhere. Since my stiffness and soreness had accompanied me on my endeavor, the stretching and twisting of my body hurt and inspired me to crankiness. After spending far too much time in the depths of the "contortium," I deduced that the dashboard had to be moved out of the way to access the modular duct. My body said, "No, you will not contort me anymore." So, after a rest, I forced myself to put the pieces back on the dash and took the torture chamber to a shop. I hadn't even dismantled enough stuff to reveal the part the book described!

I left it at my favorite mechanic shop for repair. Although, I knew I could do the job. I deemed wrenching my body into grotesque shapes in order to do so as self-inflicted stupidity. I grumbled about it as ka-ching sounds seemed to be back-masked within the everyday sounds of life. The shop completed the project by the end of the day. I had made the right decision, but didn't like it.

Later, I stood at the counter to pay for the services rendered when the mechanic that worked on it walked in. He then began a blow-by-blow dissertation of the battle he had fought to replace the heater core. He related he had to sit upside down in the seat to access the project. It seems he had to remove the bolts holding the dash in place to get at the heater core. Really? The book didn't say so. What a surprise!

Once he had removed the plastic cover, loosened the dashboard, and moved it enough to access the stuff stuffed under it, he discovered that there wasn't any modular duct at all. I surmise that the dashboard got in the way of the assembler at the factory, so for the sake of time, he hid it somewhere and went on to the next vehicle. The mechanic continued on about how he had to call around to salvage yards and secure one for the paltry sum of $60.00. (I fussed that I could have gotten one at a pull-it-yourself type of salvage yard for a fraction of that cost. But my body voiced its opposition to such an idea, "What makes you think you could get one out of a vehicle there when you couldn't at home?" I gave in to my PD, once again).

The tech demonstrated the contortions he had gone through to reach the bolts and such, which almost brought tears to my eyes as I thought about trying to do such activity. After he finished his discourse, complete with personal opinions tossed in for free, I told him that that is why I hired him – he got paid to spend time in the "contortium."

The idea of a Parkinsonian contortionist is a figment of some demented mind or else the feeble attempt of a "Parkie" to cling to his waning physical abilities. If he insists on proving that he is still able to do what he used to, just let him spend some time in a "contortium" and he will learn to behave himself. I did.

Change Changes Things

Don't you just love change? Some changes are good, like enhancing your image with a new car complete with that new car smell. Driving down the street with new flair and vitality, what is better? Except when you have someone riding with you and they want the radio, heater or air conditioner turned on. Then all you can think of is how the controls worked on your previous vehicle. But the new car is different, they changed it! Aliens from Mars or "Iowegians" must have designed it. It smacks vehemently against masculine pride to pull over, get out the owner's manual and look it up. This means coming to an "all stop" just because someone changed something. Argh. Don't you just love change?

PD has brought many changes into my life. I looked it up in Webster's and one of the definitions for "change" is that things are out of whack, which begs the question when is something in whack? Change itself, then, is whack. Since PD brought change, my life has been out of whack; thus, PD is whacky. I resent change.

I used to be a real "zoomster" filled with boundless energy. Now I move in slow motion. Prior to PD the days never had enough time to accomplish everything. Then I would think of more things to do and try to get them all done, too. PD changed that. Many times I must push myself just to go forward. I must make myself do stuff. However, I have learned that if I don't get it all done today, there is always tomorrow. I am not part of the Procrastinators Guild. I just need to rest at times. I discovered that the project does not need to be finished before I go to bed, and my bed may call out to me at any time during the day. My pillow loves me. My bed can feel like a loving, benevolent friend there to comfort me and give me rest whenever I need it. But my bed doesn't help me get things done, so I cannot reside there. Change can be frustrating.

I've heard it said that PD doesn't affect the thinking. I must disagree. I think in slow motion, one topic at a time. Remember the old eight-ball toys that you roll over and look in the little window and a word would float up? That's how my mind works now. Sometimes I can't think of a word - that is the purpose of a thesaurus. Some writers and speakers think synonyms are for variety, but the reality is that synonyms are equivalents to insert when another word is playing hide-and-seek in the recesses of my mind. Change can be mind-numbing.

PD has a penchant to pummel the male ego (definitely one of those "out of whack" things). On the occasions that I cannot open a jar, or win the struggle with a zip lock bag, or untwist a twisty on the loaf of bread, I delegate the hindrance to my wife. By considering it a delegation, it isn't a failure in manliness, I simply allowed someone else to do it, which just happens to be my wife. If I'd allow my manly pride to dictate, I'd end up losing the battle to some defiant container in a spectacular but humiliating manner. For example, we buy the plastic bags of frosted flakes. All one is supposed to do is tear the strip off the top of the new bag and then pull apart the zip lock portion and pour out the cereal. However, on one occasion I pulled the strip off in pieces, and began trying to pull apart the zip lock portion. It decided to be difficult, so I had to increase the pulling action until grunting sounds and gritting teeth showed up, but to no avail. Every man knows that a sudden sharp application of force is more effective than steady pressure. Consequently, I knew a good jerk should part the plastic and this I did – too hard! The bag split from top to bottom and the kitchen floor received a nice coating of flakiness. Change can be humiliating.

When one enters the backdoor of my house, a dark stairway lurks like a hungry vortex waiting to pull me down it once again. After my life changing injury of falling down the stairs and herniating a disc in my back, my wife asked if I was now ready to move our bedroom and "office" from the basement to the main level in order to minimize the number of my excursions up and down the stairway. I had to change my thinking, because this modification was an admission of weakness. I thereby consoled myself with the fact that we were not moving a hospital bed into the living room, so no big deal. A change for the better, I must admit, but an even better one would be to move into a lovely one level home without the animosity of stairways lying in wait to nab me. Things keep changing.

The change from working a job everyday, to being unable to do such a job ever again meant admitting defeat to PD once again.

At the time of this writing, my back is much improved, but the PD took advantage of its opportunity to gain ground. It had already eroded my ability to "hobbyshop" on cars, but now my stamina fell victim, as well. My quads have not returned to the point of dependability, so I must use a cane. I changed my thinking and decided a cane is not an old man's support system, but a stylish augmentation to my daily ensemble.

Change changes things.

Sleep Interrupted

I like dreams, at least most of them. As a youngster, daydreams occupied my imagination. But nowadays reality steps in and squashes them like a tennis shoe dispatching an ant. Once in a while a good idea slips through and I entertain it for a while, but all in all, I don't dream like I used to. I had a flash of genius once, but it zipped through my consciousness with the sound and speed of an Indy style race car, too fast to grasp, and disappeared. However, it's the dreams that I can't control that bother me. They interrupt my sleep.

I took a nap the other day. Since I was unconscious at the time, I missed most of it, but I do remember a negative event during said siesta. My subconscious mind ran amuck without my permission and I found my sleep interrupted. Experience has taught me that a nice peaceful snooze can be ruined by alarm clocks, telephones, Harley Davidson motorcycles, thunder and an occasional nightmare. I can blame most of those things on someone else, but not the nightmares. They are self-produced scariness – not that I am out to scare myself, I just do, which displeases me immensely. I am happy that most times I forget the fright within minutes of waking up.

The ones I remember, though, usually have to do with bees. I don't know why. As a kid, I used to catch them for fun. They have earned my respect by stinging me a few times, but I do not have an irrational fear of them. I enjoy honey, yet don't overindulge, so that can't be it. I even had a run-in on our trip to Malawi with African honeybees – those that look like our honeybees, but have a bad attitude. While the exterminators did their thing, I stood nearby with a camera fearlessly photographing the entire episode.

The only disturbing experience regarding stinging insects that I remember was the episode of yellow jackets that had commandeered a wall of a garage we had in Idaho. A previous owner had put paneling on the interior of the storeroom on the north end, which created a well-appreciated barrier between me and the bugs. But on a hot summer day I could hear the "bzzzz" without putting my ear to the wall, and could also smell an odd sickening odor. I imagined thousands of yellow jackets in there building housing for still more little "nasties." I had observed them carrying paralyzed insects into their hive as food for the newly hatched larvae. This explained the strange aroma on hot days. I did find that rather creepy.

Not long after we moved there, we were stacking firewood behind the garage, near their hole-in-the-wall hideout, and we alarmed one of the lookouts – didn't know the buzzword, no doubt. My son felt the affects of the air strike. In retaliation, I plugged their holes with spray-in foam insulation, but that didn't stop them. They just chewed through and went on with life as normal. However, when I refilled their holes with insulation again and soaked that with insecticide, I won. No more "buzziness" in the wall.

This event could very well be the catalyst for my bee dreams, which always revolve around a similar theme. In my nightmares, the honeybees have build a super-hive somewhere in my house, maybe under it, in the walls, or in the attic, depending upon the dreamscape.

In one particular dream they had built such a huge hive in the attic that the honey ran down the walls to the level below and caused the ceiling to bow downward. From the outside, I could see thousands of bees coming and going through a one foot square attic vent, located immediately under the point of the roof of the old house. Obviously, they had been there for years, and coexisted peacefully with the previous tenants, but now something had to be done.

I opened the access hole to the attic and a very loud "zzzzzzzz" assaulted my ear drums causing my adrenaline to flow freely and my anxiety to grow. I stuck my head up there to survey the situation. The walls were covered with honeycomb and huge stalactites and stalagmites of the stuff filled the room. Bees flew everywhere busily busy with whatever bees do. I had heard how bees tell other bees where to find honey. It only made sense that they would relay information regarding intruders, as well. So, I slowly dropped back down, hoping they hadn't noticed me. I woke up without resolution of the problem.

The nightmare always consists of me attempting to deal with this dilemma. I try various things, and seek advice from other people. I try smoking them out with some kind of smoke producing gadget, playing awful rock music to drive them out, spraying cans of bug fumigator, or firing a "buzzooka" but nothing works. The only thing I accomplish is to wake up anxious and frustrated. I don't go back to sleep easily because the dream doesn't dissipate from my memory like other dreams.

I don't know whether I can blame such dreams on Parkinson's, but many Parkies do have nightmares. I am also unsure as to whether my dreams rate up there with true horror or not, but they certainly are not something I would consciously dream up and inflict upon myself.

I prefer my sleep to remain uninterrupted – I hope the bees won't buzz me during nap times in the future.

Spinning Out of Control

I decided to help my physical rehabilitation, physical appearance, and general physicality by buying a stationary bike. The recumbent variety looked more appealing than the upright – that should be reserved for real bicycling. This one doesn't have any bells and whistles, but it does have a cool instrument cluster, well it actually has only one display screen, but it tells you many things, like the RPM's, speed, time and distance. The RPM's vary a lot depending upon on how fast I am pedaling. The timer works sporadically. At times it goes really fast and I'm done quickly, but when I really don't feel like pedaling, it goes slower. My heart rate, according to its sensor, can vary from 89 to 150 at the beginning of my workout and at the end, either my heart has a problem or the bike lies. I opt for the dishonesty of the bike.

It also has a couple of courses I could go on. The graph shows hills and valleys, but even if I close my eyes and use my imagination, I don't notice the hills or valleys. Instead it contains a "nagivator" option with idiot lights that say "go faster" or "go slower." Perhaps if I read the book, things would make more sense, but if that got out I might receive hate mail from various men's groups for actually reading an owner's manual.

The recumbent aspect is cool except for one thing. The seam of my jeans lines up perfectly with my tailbone, which after vigorous activity can leave a blister. How do you explain to people that you can't sit down because you have a blister on your tailbone? They either doubt your sanity or they think it's really from watching too much TV. They may even think it is a bed sore from lazing around all day.

I like the appearance of the bike. It has a sporty streamlined look as if wind resistance was an issue. And it has a wide stance and low center of gravity, perfect for cornering. Not to mention the trick paint job. Another feature is that if I decide to stop, I stop, no problem, not like a treadmill which will keep going, pull my feet out from under me and scrape skin off my nose. Nope, I'll stick to my bike.

The bike also has these nifty stirrups that are designed to hold my feet on the pedals at high speeds. However, they are merely marketing gimmicks, because at high speed, which doesn't happen often, my feet fly out, my knees hit the handle bars and then my feet smack the floor while the pedals flail at my thighs. Not a pleasant experience. Maybe duct tape would work better than their designer toe clamps. (Red Green would be proud).

I recently discovered that stationary bicycling is a sport of sorts and has been renamed spinning. I thought that was a precursor to quilting or knitting. Then again since it was in a health facility, it could have been something like a whirling dervish. I could join such a group, but I would have to get a firm grasp on the controls or I would be definitely spinning out of control.

My Personal Trainer

Whoever heard of a Baptist preacher, retired or otherwise, having a personal trainer? He's the kind that trains the client right in his own home. Believe it or not, I have one, and he is tough!

He came into my life in July of 2010. I had injured my back and lost my job, plus dealing with Parkinson's disease – a time when I really needed one. I still utilize his services on a daily basis, because his antics and drive have helped muchly.

First thing in the morning, he arrives with enough energy to power a city of 100,000 for a week. I really like him, but his cheerful enthusiasm can drive me crazy, especially on a bad day, similar to the idea expressed in Proverbs 27:14 *He that blesseth his friend with a loud voice, rising early in the morning, it shall be counted a curse to him.* I used to wake up with that kind of energy, but my Parkinson's has stolen that. He acts like his energy will rub off on me, thus enabling me to endure the rigors of physical activity. The reality is that his youth and vitality make me feel old and out of shape.

He sports one of those popular hairstyles that make him look like he just crawled out of bed. Certainly, he doesn't spend time in front of the mirror purposefully "disasterizing" his hair with an electric mixer, but it makes one wonder. However, for good trainer/client relationship, he does try to please me and has made efforts to allow someone to tame his hair, although it doesn't last long. Maybe it is a naturally occurring phenomenon.

I generally feed him breakfast, in order to build rapport. After which, I begin my workout by stretching my muscles. He advocates the importance of routine – that is doing the same things in the same order at the same time every day. If I slack off by getting off schedule, he fusses and nags me to buckle down - we must stick to routine.

Parkinson's disease can make my muscles stiff and sore, especially on bad days. He makes me stretch them anyway! My trainer wants me to stretch the tight muscles that bring my shoulders forward and cause my back to stoop. He gives little vocalizations to "press on" as I grimace at the discomfort.

To stretch my quads, I stand against the arm of the couch so I don't tip over, and pull my right foot up toward my derrière. At this point, my trainer has situated himself on the couch and voices some inspirational utterances, while I complain about the soreness. Next, I stretch out one leg at a time behind me and work on the calves, with him checking carefully that I am doing it correctly. Then I put a foot up on the arm of the couch and gently touch my toe, with him watching carefully that my fingers actually touch and making sure I do both legs, as well. He believes I should have caught up to his drive and ambition by this point.

Then my trainer meets me in the middle of the living room floor. He is so energetic! I lie on my stomach and arc my back by pushing up with my arms and keeping my hips on the floor. Since I am on the floor, my coach gets in my face to push me to do pushups. He counts each one and checks to make sure I execute full pushups as well as making it slow and deliberate for a good squeeze on the muscles. Coach, a true motivational speaker, pushes me on – he can be so mean! Once I had to tell him to get off my back, literally – he had crossed the line that time.

My personal trainer also has me roll over and stretch my lower back by pulling my knees up to my chest and holding. If I take a moment to relax he gets after me immediately. I then twist my legs to the right and to the left. My personal trainer puts his nose to the floor to check out that my legs actually make contact with the floor. I then do some other stretches while my coach keeps an eye on my progress. Since I am on my back on the floor, he has me execute some sit-ups. He flits about from floor level, to standing, to perching in a chair, all the while prodding me to keep going. He rivals the annoyance level of Richard Simmons.

Coach has me go to a chair and stand up and sit down several times to strengthen my thighs. He would spur me on with real spurs, if he could. His enthusiastic friskiness is supposed to stimulate my adrenal glands – supposed to…

I'm glad that my coach didn't view the video I saw at a Parkinson's disease conference in April, 2010. It showed a rat on miniature treadmill, but he didn't want to walk because he had a drug-induced form of Parkinson's. The base of the treadmill had an electric grid - if he didn't walk he would fall off the end and receive a shock. What a motivator! My coach would love to have a tazer set on "move it" to prompt me into action with an electrical shock when I slow down.

When nasty weather, of one form or another, prevents

outside activities, I ride my recumbent stationary bike. I read a book or pray while I pedal; coach doesn't and struggles with boredom. He has even fallen asleep. I chide him about it, a couple of times I have even yelled out in a loud and abrupt manner, which startles him and entertains me.

After finishing my stretches and exercises, he goes to my closet and points out my walking shoes – as if I need to be told which pair of shoes to wear! I grab my cane, and we go outside for a 20-30 minute walk. He pushes for a fast pace. But he gets what I can give. If I am slow he tugs on his leash and looks back at me as if to say, "Well, are we gonna walk or what?" Once we have returned to the house he shows off by running laps around the house.

The name on his "business card" is: T. Bone Dickens, or Dickens for short. By including my Yorkshire Terrier in my daily regiment, I inadvertently trained him to be my personal trainer. The idea for his name is that he is cute as the dickens. However, as a personal trainer he can be quite the dickens.

Sudoku-ku

Every once in a while my wife would try to teach me Sudoku. It is a puzzle found next to the crossword puzzle in our newspaper. It is a box containing smaller boxes which hold even smaller boxes looking similar to a sketch of a waffle iron grid. The idea is to fill those little boxes with numbers. That is where the problem comes in. A crossword puzzle makes sense because when letters, which represent sounds, are put in a certain order they make words. The same letters can be rearranged to make new words. By just making the sounds of the letters a word can be sounded out. On the other hand, the arrangement of numbers makes no difference. Numbers have been a bane to me all my life, especially now with PD. But, since it is important to use my gray matter I decided to learn how to do Sudoku. The directions in a puzzle book said:

To solve a Sudoku puzzle, place a number into each box so that each row across, each column down, and each small 9-box square within the larger diagram (there are 9 of these) will contain every number from 1 through 9. In other words, no number may appear more than once in any row, column, or smaller 9-box square. Working with the numbers already given as a guide, complete each diagram with the missing numbers that will lead to the correct solution.

Reading that didn't help me understand it one bit. So,

my wife reiterated the entire instructions, which went in one ear and got stuck somewhere inside. I heard Katie say stuff like, "This row contains all the numbers which cannot be repeated."

Me: "Ok, I can understand that."

Katie: "Then this column contains all the numbers too, which cannot be repeated."

Me: "But they share a number, right?"

Katie: "Right.

Me: "But they cannot be repeated, right?"

Katie: "Right, now you're getting it."

Me: "I hear a strange sound like a needle scratching across a phonograph record."

Katie: "Now see this square?"

Me: "I see lots of squares."

Katie: "I know, but see this square that contains nine smaller squares?

Me: "Yup."

Katie: "Well, that contains all the numbers, which cannot be repeated, too."

Me: "Huh?"

Katie: "You see, this box contains......" And the words she said began bumping into one another causing a verbal traffic jam in my head.

Me: "My brain can't take this. I need to take a break before it gets bruised."

Katie: "Ok, take a breather…now try to fill in this number."

Me: "We are going to have to take my brain in for treatment of contusions and abrasions."

Katie: "Just try this one right here."

Me: "I think I feel a hemorrhage taking place."

Katie: "Sudoku has never killed anyone."

Me: "Are you sure? Maybe it is just causing a herniation, like my back injury."

Katie: "You'll be fine."

Me: "I can't even pronounce it the same way consistently. The syllables don't roll off the tongue. This whole thing is driving me cuckoo."

Katie: "Sudoku-ku, cuckoo, cuckoo."

Me: "Hey that can help me remember how to say it!"

Regardless of my protests and objections, Katie patiently coached me through several puzzles. Then on December 8, 2010 I conquered Sudoku! I actually finished two games, with my wife's supervision. I even soloed on the easiest level several times since then – without supervision! I can't imagine attempting to solve the hardest level without causing severe lacerations of the basal ganglia, which, in turn, would result in dopamine leakage.

I've heard much about the idea that exercising helps the brain as well as the brawn. So, I do stretches and ride my stationary bike every day and walk when weather permits, as well. The puzzling thing is how much sudoku is beneficial and how much is detrimental. So, if you see me one day with my head in a sling, you'll know I sprained my brain puzzling over those number grids.

Raising Cane

I discovered in a rather rude abrupt manner the unforgiving and abrasive nature of concrete. It leaves marks upon one's body if given the opportunity. Whether it's less embarrassing to sport a cane or to display marks that lead to inquiries is the question. I chose to sport a cane.

During a night in July of 2010, I descended our darkened stairway in an unexpected and ungraceful manner during the wee hours of the morning. Things went amiss and amuck, and I somehow landed on my tailbone and continued thumping my way down in an ungainly twisting fashion until I stopped on the carpeted concrete floor. My lower back hurt somewhat, but I went to bed thinking I had survived without any visible discoloration or disfigurement to explain to my family at breakfast in the morning. Even though the pain didn't subside during the week, I went to work anyway. Throughout this time the lack of support from our super-soft pillow-top mattress contributed to the injury and rendered me unable to work the following week. During the second week, I twisted in a way that pinched the nerve and I discovered what a 10 rating of pain really felt like. I found myself lying on the floor, making noises that caused our new puppy to express his concern vocally and summoned the cat over to lay paws on me, similar to that of a faith healer. Since her spirituality is seriously lacking, her efforts did not help.

The injury caused my quads (the front area of the thighs) on my right leg to go berserk. The muscles danced and frolicked unashamedly throughout the day and into the night; then they started the party again the next morning.

Several rounds of physical therapy and a lumbar shot ruined their hoedown and calmed them tremendously. However, the quads have never returned to their pre-injury status. To this day, the muscles will occasionally decide to wake me up at night by spastic behavior, which sends me into action to alleviate the pain by rubbing the muscles, stretching (if possible), using the vibrator and heating pad. After their spasmodic conduct has abated, sleep is slow to return. Nothing wakes up a man like pain. Even on good mornings, I still must not stretch the muscles until after my morning dose of PD meds or they will begin riotous cramping and cavorting.

Since my injury (and perhaps before – maybe that was the cause of my stairwell descension) my quads will let me down, literally. I can walk 50, 75, 100 steps or more, then without warning they will take a break and the ground will jump up to hit some portion of my anatomy. This triggers an unwanted hubbub with nearby people and colors me embarrassing hues of pink and red. Sometimes I display an abrasion for a few days, which prompts questions or suppositions that my wife has been mean to me. As a result, I sport a cane. I try not to lean on the cane, but simply use it as a stabilizing stick when the quads cease and desist from doing their job.

Walmart knew I would need a cane and stocked some just for me. I found one that could be broken down and stuffed into a suitcase if necessary. Think about it, a collapsible cane. Sounds dangerous, but that is what I came home with. Someday I plan to acquire a designer cane, one of those full of cool twists and gnarls with Psalm 17:5 somehow engraved on it: *"Hold up my goings in thy paths, that my footsteps slip not."*

When I go for a walk, now with my collapsible cane, endorphins somewhere along the way hitchhike with me for a while. I enjoy them, even though I don't see them. My theory is that flocks of them hide in the trees and drop down on my head as I pass by. I never notice them, I just realize I feel better and, thusly, understand and appreciate the fact that I have encountered them. They prove better than a sunrise or birds singing in the morning because they don't just encourage, they actually make me feel better. They have less chance to hop on board these days as I used to walk one or two miles. At the time of this writing, it is just around the block before the quads start becoming unstable or begin dancing. My neurologist says the problem with the quads is the back injury and the spinal specialist feels it is the Parkinson's. I think it is a combination thereof. But, what to do? I sport a cane.

Now, I am stylin' like Mr. Peanut on the Planters Peanuts label - although, I can't see myself in the top hat and monocle. How does one keep the monocle in place, scrunch up your face constantly? That would require concentration that I need for timing the cane with my steps. How about wearing a bowler like Charlie Chaplin? Perhaps, but swinging the cane around like he did just seems like a disaster in the making and misadventures like me anyway, so why attract them. I simply think of my cane as an image enhancer and a thwarter of embarrassment when used properly.

When I began sporting a cane, I discovered that the

talent of juggling would be a help. Whenever I purchase something at a store, I must lean the cane up against the counter or my leg in order to free both hands to conduct the transaction. I have tried pressing it tightly against the counter or jamming it into my car keys or wallet nestled in my pocket, but nothing works. Once I have both hands full the cane always starts to fall. All I can do is simply stand there and watch the cane fall – all the way to the floor! Argh. But then if it wasn't for the floor it would still be falling, so I shouldn't fuss so much. I have wondered if a string fastened on it like a yo-yo would help; when it falls just snap it back up. Then I think of being tethered to a stick and realize that more problems exist where there are strings attached.

Because of my back injury, sitting for a period of time has proved difficult for a few months. Consequently, we sat in the rear of the church so that I could slip out quietly and stand in the back of the auditorium. No problem, until one Sunday my cane escaped my grip. I unsuccessfully tried to grab it. It plummeted downward in slow motion directly toward a one-inch wide metal strip that encased the glass adjoining the glass auditorium doors. Noooooo! Why not hit the carpet? Why hit the only metal thing within reach? As the teacher of the class waxed eloquent the cane made contact abruptly with a loud metallic WHACK that woke up those dozing, and distracted the attentive ones. Heads throughout the congregation pivoted and fixed their gaze on me as I picked up my cane.   At that point, I realized I had just raised cane in church. But I still sport a cane.

Work, a Spectator Sport

Katie says I drive like an old man nowadays. She may be right. As a teen, I remember my dad complaining about driving in the snow, but I found excitement in it. Getting stuck? Adventure! No travel advised? That was no warning, it was a dare. But now such a hazardous undertaking has relinquished itself to a bother of exceeding aggravation. The whole procedure exacerbates the stiffness, soreness, and fatigue which robs me of the reward of adventure. So, it's better to watch adventures from the window than to participate.

I have discovered that PD is a great male ego deflater. In many ways I have turned into a "use-ta-wasser." I *use to* do a lot of stuff I *was* able to do that is no longer possible. Now when snow starts to fall I sound like…horrors, my father!

In past years I and my son, had experienced the adventurous activity of clearing the sidewalk and driveway. But since my son has moved into his own apartment, Katie has gotten the privilege of running the snow blower. She, somehow, does not appreciate the experience of firing up a machine, feeling the vibration of the motor and getting a thrill out of it. She says that it is noisy and stinks. That's all she gets out of it? For some unknown reason, she simply does not enjoy the exhilaration of snow blowing back in her face, nor does she relish the frigid temps in general. I witness the adventure from the warmth of the living room, but it frustrates me to see her experiencing the exhilaration meant for me!

At the time of this writing, we just received meteorological nastiness consisting of rain, freezing rain, sleet and a combination thereof which built up a respectable layer of frozen stuff all over – even surfaces that demand removal of said iciness. This two inch layer proved a formidable opponent in the snow removal process requiring a tedious chipping procedure. Since the cleanup was especially stubborn I asked the teen group from our church to come and whittle, scrape, shovel, and thus remove the frozen crust from our concrete surfaces.

The neighbor across the street unknowingly provided entertainment to help me pass the time until the teens arrived. He, obviously not a local, tried to get his old Chevy van to go uphill by pushing the accelerator down and letting the tires burn down through the two-inch layer of ice as smoke and steam drifted upward. He would get out and dig, climb back in, produce smoke and steam, get out and dig, get back in and create another cloud of white and bluish steam. The rear wheels contributed to the rising vapor, as well. A little patience, sand, and shifting into reverse would have solved their problem. I debated whether to risk being viewed as a know-it-all by going out there and volunteering my knowledge. However, another risk would be getting stuck helping him get unstuck by digging and pushing – something my body would complain about for days. So, I stayed in the house and looked out the window – like an old man!

Then the story began to build. Another neighbor hooked up a tow rope to his four-wheel-drive Dodge pickup and tried to pull the van uphill. The Ram-tough pickup had all four wheels spinning, throwing rooster-tails of white stuff at the van while steam still rose from the van, as well.

About that time the plot thickened - a snowplow came along. It just couldn't get any better! He waited for a minute or two while the four-wheeler tried his best to move the van. Then he decided to try pulling it downhill, so the plow lifted his blade, leaving a pile of snow behind the van and continued on his way.

The action sequence consisted of the Dodge's four tires spinning just as futilely as before. I told the driver of the van to shift it out of park, but he couldn't hear my advice due to the sound deadening qualities of a picture window in the way. Eventually, he figured it out himself. I seriously wanted to dash out there, like a volunteer neighborhood watchman and advisor, to recommend the van driver straighten his wheels since he still had the wheels pointed sharply left. But I knew I would never make it in time. Besides, it would have ruined the show.

Once the Dodge broke the Chevy loose, it swung up onto the old crusty snow piles! Its predicament had worsened. It now leaned at a twenty-degree angle jammed onto the berm. The Dodge spun four rooster-tails into the air, stopped, backed up and zoomed until he hit the end of the tow rope, which pulled the van higher onto the wall of frozen plow deposits. After several runs, the driver walked back to the driver of the Chevy van, motioned to him vigorously to straighten his wheels and tried again. "Wala-tada" the Chevy dropped off the snow bank!

What a climactic let-down! The show was over. The epilogue consisted of the van driver utilizing the same winter driving techniques that got him into his predicament in the first place, as he reattempted to ascend the hill while the four-by-four went home. I made a great spectator, giving unheard advice and all.

I then looked out the window to check on my elderly neighbor lady next door still chipping away at the frozen mess. I wanted to help, but realized that I could not do as much as she could, argh!

Then it hit me, maybe I have turned into an old man because such adventures have now become a spectator sport.

"Bleepazoids"

I must preface this essay by saying that most people I meet are decent and helpful, but unfortunately, one also meets "bleepazoids." They come in assorted shapes and sizes, as well as in every age group. Recently I met a couple of extraordinarily accomplished "bleepazoids" that took an opportunity to increase the stress factor in the area immediately surrounding them - Bermuda Triangle I happened to wander into.

After parking my Sonoma, I walked across the parking lot toward the front door of a store. I felt good and was enjoying the day. As I neared the entrance, I noticed a man standing by a piece of furniture, waiting for a vehicle to arrive for loading. Just as I started crossing the main thoroughfare of the parking lot, a small station wagon pulled up within a couple feet of me and blocked my trajectory toward the front door. So, I stopped. The male "bleepazoid" let loose a string of profanity aimed at the driver for nearly driving over his foot. A young woman appeared behind the car, as the man continued swearing at the kids to stay in the car and then again at the driver for nearly running over his foot.

Since the car remained in a stationary position, I started around the front of it, as it started moving forward. I stopped. It stopped. I stepped forward. It started moving. I stopped. It stopped. I started moving. It started moving. I stopped and said to myself, "Well, what are we doing?" while I inadvertently made a small open-handed gesture with my hands (meaning, "I don't know what to do because I don't know what you are going to do). I was not upset, angry, perturbed, or in any other way feeling negatively about this event. I was simply unsure of whether to take another step or not.

Suddenly a different voice screeched through the air, "Chill, (bleeeep)." A female "bleepazoid!"

"I'm sorry, did I do something?" I asked, thinking surely she couldn't be upset with me, yet speaking to her because she seemed intent on glaring at me.

She began a tirade so filled with profanity and name calling that she could have saved a lot of wear and tear on her vocal chords if she had omitted them. In short, this was no "bleepazoidian" slip.

"I didn't know what they were going to do?" I responded.

She asked me, with the grace and benevolence of a badger vexed with an unmentionable physical malady, exactly what did I think they were doing. Her question included adjectives not found in any reputable dictionary.

I responded that I honestly didn't know because they had stopped and resumed forward motion three times.

The male bleepaziod, who obviously had never heard of Dale Carnegie's book on making friends and influencing people, entered the fray by demanding from the female, what the problem was.

That revved her up tremendously. As she informed him, her voice grew in volume and intensity until it could compete with feedback in any amplification system. She then shifted into animation mode. She proceeded to demonstrate an extremely exaggerated version of my inadvertent hand movement and said "He went like this".

She then turned to me and said that she had never met such a (an assortment of expletives deleted) in all her life!

I wanted to think that he was afraid of contradicting her to avoid her wrath spewing forth in his direction, but drawing from his earlier diatribe at those in the car, he obviously thought much like she did. The male "bleepazoid" turned to me and yelled, "Why don't you take your crippled (bleep) home and get out of our way?"

I asked if he was kidding, and wondered how this could be a problem for them. My astonishment orbited my amazement as I made a wide arc behind the vehicle and made my way to the door situated immediately on the other side of the car. I endured a barrage of profanity and insults as they set the public relations example for their kids. They railed about never meeting such a (bleep) in all their lives and how cripples were (unrepeatable names).

I hunkered down and headed for the store entrance as the obscenities splattered against the glass doors like rain, hail and wind in a thunderstorm. Once safe inside from the vulgarity storm, I walked the aisles trying to determine whether that had really happened! The stress intensified my tremor, my emotions and the cognitive aspects of PD. By talking with my wife on the phone and hearing her calm reassuring words, I got where I could function again.

Stressful episodes of this intense nature are harder to deal with than they were prior to PD.

Waxed to the Max

In 2010, my Dad and I attended Automania[2] at the Sioux Empire fairgrounds in Sioux Falls, SD. As I drove through the entrance in my 1992 GMC Sonoma, an official looking guy started giving me directions to park, as if I had entered it in the show. My ego grew a bit, but an inflating ego sucks the oxygen from the immediate area, and causes yawning amongst others. So, keeping my ego in check is a must. Besides I dislike the humiliation when God deflates it.

At this point, my old dream of owning a bona fide show car fluttered to the surface of my dreamscape, but reality quickly shot it down. Since PD came along, I am unable to build such a car anymore, plus the financial aspect to simply purchase a nice rod looked bleak.

Automania 2011 spurred this idea again, but with a twist to the dream. Why not show the Sonoma, while you still can? After all, I told myself, it's about twenty years old and looks sharp enough to spur compliments from people younger than the truck (anything built after the year one is born is not old; its simply getting rare). Since it is my daily transportation it is not really nice enough to show. However, while attending a NPF/SD event at a local retirement home, I discovered that they were sponsoring a car show for the residents in the near future. Since they did not charge a registration fee, and in fact, bribed the participants with a free dinner, I signed up – at the last moment! I justified my decision by telling myself that I could at least help fill the parking lot for the residents. Suddenly, I realized I was

---

[2] An annual car show in Sioux Falls, SD

committed, or perhaps, should have been committed to a mental institution.

Even though I generally kept it clean and waxed, preparations were in order. I worked away at it sporadically, over the limited time I had to spiff it up. I began by picking up some polish, wax and also some degreaser for under the hood. I applied the degreaser, let it sit for the required time and then grabbed the hose - which I accidentally dropped on the driveway. The little gun let loose in my face, and wouldn't let up until I had fought my way upstream, ambushed it and squelched its little game. Eventually, I transferred the grease from the vehicle to me and our concrete driveway.

I had always wondered what kind of nut it took to clean a car with a toothbrush – until I found myself using one to scrub the crevasses around the hoses, air cleaner, radiator shroud, wires, cables and other miscellaneous things. I even waxed some of the parts! Who waxes under the hood? The same kind of nut that scrubs his car with a toothbrush, that's who. As this process began feeling like vehicular worship and therefore, lunacy, my PD rose up and declared the area under the hood, "good enough."

On another day, I moved on to the exterior, scrubbed the box clean, and waxed the rest, grudgingly including the wheels. It took only a few minutes to clean and apply ArmorAll to the interior. I praised God for the small pickup cab and not the expanse of a station wagon! I even cleaned the door hinges – with that vile toothbrush! By the time I had finished, I had used enough shop towels, terry cloth towels, cotton rags and work clothes to fill the washing machine. I had waxed weary of being a nut with a soapy toothbrush and a rag hanging out my back pocket, Gomer-style and said, "Enough of this nonsense!" Besides my PD had had enough and let me know it, through great stiffness, soreness and bone-tired fatigue.

I still had a problem, though. Some parking lot bozo had backed up until they hit something and then left - my grill, in pieces. I called several salvage yards. One local auto recycler said they had one in good condition. I went to see if I and the counterman agreed on the meaning of "good condition". As I walked in, the two countermen and a customer were so intensely engaged in conversation that they barely acknowledged my arrival. Eventually, a lull in the conversation that lasted well beyond awkward occurred. One of them looked in my direction and, with all the cheerfulness of a bored old bloodhound on a hot day, said, "Yeah?"

I considered this my cue and related the phone conversation I had earlier with an unnamed counterman. The second counterman on duty turned to his computer in an obligatory manner and clicked away at the keyboard. Without looking up from the screen, he asked no one in particular if a Jimmy and a Sonoma grill interchanged. Counterman One said, "Yup." Counterman Two scribbled something on a piece of paper. He then gave it to an employee that had wandered in. He left, leaving the awkward atmosphere to hang like an unidentifiable odor, while he wandered the organized chaos of parts in search of the grill. I began to wonder if he had killed time, because it wasn't showing signs of movement anymore. Eventually, he returned with a grill. It looked good, so I bought it and let the conversationalists return to their previous discourse. It took longer to clean up the grill than to install it, but the counterman had been right, it did look good.

On the humorous side, I could joke with others that I had wanted a new grill for Father's Day, and ended up buying it for myself – from an auto salvage yard!

Finally, the day of the show arrived. Katie and I drove up a little early to secure a good place to park. I noticed a spot between an El Camino and an International pickup and parked between them. Upon registration I received a ticket for my free meal and bought Katie a meal, as well. I had offered to let her drive, so she could get the free meal, but she either felt more honored and special if I bought her meal or, more likely, she wanted me to get the glory of driving an old pickup truck around. A third option crossed my mind – that only I get the free meal - which I dismissed quickly. I'm not necessarily the brightest bulb on the Christmas Tree, but I had learned something, eating in front of one's wife without getting her anything was not the wisest option – even if she says its not a problem.

At this point, we realized that other participants had claimed the shady spots, sat in their own lawn chairs and watched other people, who sat in lawn chairs and watched them. We did not bring lawn chairs and so we had to sit directly on the grass – no problem if you are young and agile, because getting down was much easier than getting up again.

After a short time, the retirement home started serving the appropriate drive-up fare of barbecued burgers, shakes, fries and soda pop. They had even recruited the local roller derby girls as car hops, although everybody sat at tables or in their lawn chairs.   While they ate, many people told car related stories, including some that had obviously been waxed and polished as much as their cars.

My Sonoma turned out to be the newest of the old cars – if you didn't count the late model four-door Mercury sedan. The other cars drew much more attention, but my Sonoma added some color and chrome to the event. My desire to show a car waxed to the max has now waned to the point that I again wonder about people who clean their cars with a toothbrush. Waxing to the max is more taxing than I ever want to do again.

If I ever actually write out my "bucket list," I can immediately cross off, "car show." Reason and the reality of life with Parkinson's has returned!

"Appy" Day

"What a way to spend a Sunday," I said to myself as I thought back on the day before (my Sundays always revolved around church – especially since I was pastor of a church in North Idaho at the time). As the previous Saturday had progressed, I began to feel sick. By the time Katie had gotten off work, I had spent much of my time in the bathroom. Plus, a pain element had begun to intensify to the point of misery. However, since such disturbances can usually be attributed to obnoxious food behavior, we decided to see how it went through the night. Sleep came but didn't overstay its welcome. By sunrise, the pain had worsened. Katie made a phone call to a nurse friend that urgently implored that we get to the emergency room ASAP. In her opinion it could be appendicitis and, therefore, even though it was Sunday medical attention should not be delayed. Therefore, we put the services in the hands of our teenage son and daughter, and braved bouncy I-90 to the hospital forty-five minutes away.

Without hesitation they placed me in a wheelchair and escorted me to my own private room in the Emergency department while Katie filled out paperwork. Then I answered questions and felt like the Pillsbury Doughboy as different nurses, assistants, doctors and other people with white coats poked and prodded my abdomen. After some tests, discussion and further examination by the various hospital personnel, appendicitis was, indeed, decided upon.

The surgeon explained the needed procedure as laproscopic surgery. The "appy," as he called it, would be done through a hole he would bore through my belly button and two other holes in my abdomen. He explained that they would also fill me with hot air - wait a minute, as a preacher I have already been accused of being that! Off I went to surgery on a gurney, chatting with the anesthesiologist on the way about adverse reactions to anesthesia, allergies and the like.

Once in the operating room I found myself surrounded by people in light blue disguises. One of them talked like I should recognize him, but they all looked the same to me. Turns out he was my surgeon. The anesthesiologist put a clear cup-like thing over my nose and mouth and said to count to ten. I never made it. The next thing I knew, the ceiling tiles were bouncing back and forth in the recovery room. The only way they would stop is if I would shut my eyes; then sleep would take over. After a while they declared me "recovered" and brought me up to a hospital room with Katie. I had made it through the "appy" hour.

After awhile the anesthesia wore off. I hurt, but not more than at the other times my Parkinson's disease acted up (although I didn't know it was PD at the time). I simply utilized my old strategy of not moving a muscle to allow the pain to subside. This was prior to the PD meds like Sinemet and Mirapex.

During recovery the nurse said, "I am surprised that you didn't ask for more pain meds."

I replied, "I am used to hurting. When I lay perfectly still it gradually abates and then I stay perfectly still to keep it that way."

"Well, you need to get up and walk." She announced.

"But, it doesn't hurt right now, why aggravate the nerve endings? If they are happy, then I am happy." However, with her persistence and assistance, I got up anyway and joined the other surgery patients walking their IV poles around the hallways. I pulled up alongside another gentleman and offered to race, but he did not have the wherewithal to do so. In retrospect, I am glad that he didn't take me up on the offer. The nursing staff would have disapproved of such behavior, and I really wasn't up to it either.

Later that Monday, they released me to my wife's care. For some reason, they insisted that I take a wheelchair ride from my third floor room to the front door. Since walking was not the pleasurable experience it usually was, I accepted the offer; maybe because I still moved slower than most turtles.

After a wait just short of long, a harmless looking little retired volunteer came to drive. "The Little Ol' Lady from Pasadena" could have been playing over the speaker system to accompany her driving technique. She took off like the roadrunner in the cartoons, setting me back in the seat and zoomed. She must have irresponsibly mixed adrenaline, caffeine and sugar just before she drove. She zigged and zagged through people in the hallway like a quarterback running for the goal. The people aware of us took evasive maneuvers to avoid contact, some of which required spontaneous contortions to do so. I thought about putting a foot or two down to stop the progress, but figured at the speed we were traveling that I'd be pulled under the chair. I imagined the three small incisions and my insides being pulled apart in the process, so I decided to concentrate on hanging on. I keenly felt every elevator threshold and seam in the flooring that we thumped over, as well as the abrupt jerking and jostling as she skirted around several obstacles.

We arrived at the front door in record time; at least, I should think she had the record. As quickly as she had arrived, she was gone. It felt similar to the sudden ending of a roller coaster ride, when all motion stops but the body isn't sure yet. Momentarily, Katie caught up with me sitting in my wheelchair, abandoned. We commented on our astonishment that there had been no mishaps, accidents or incidents through that jaunt.

She retrieved the car, helped me in and we journeyed in a sane and cautious manner back home, where I spent quality time with my bed and pillow. Oh, "appy" day.

Debatable Debris

The other day I found myself engaged in a conversation with an excessively talkative fellow. Since conversation implies that both parties contribute to the discussion, a challenge presented itself.

He talked without stopping to take a breath! I wondered if he had an intake manifold or a gill-like apparatus hidden somewhere else on his person, because the air needed for vocalizations must have a source of similar proportions to supply the demand. He talked about fishing and horses and work and his brother and his sister and his dad and this and that and etcetera, etcetera, etcetera without inhaling!

I made numerous attempts to offer what I considered to be interesting and engaging comments. However, he chatted on about a deer hitting his car and that he did not hit it, the deer did all the hitting... As he related how this buck ran out of nowhere and attacked his car, I wanted to ask him why the deer had it out for him, but could only make unintelligible utterances because my words were cut short before completion.

He carried on about the damage inflicted upon his vehicle. Since I had a similar story to relate, I tried to share it. However, his words hit my interjection head-on. He countered my attempt at conversation with increased volume and intensity, which slammed mine backwards. Had it not been for my cat-like reflexes, they would have hit my head. Instead, they splattered against the wall behind me and slid down to the floor forming a pile of "clutterized" confusion.

At one point, I thought I sensed a lull coming on and let a couple of words go, but they hit a barrage of verbiage and ended up crumpled on the floor like wads of paper. After a while the verbal carnage filled the area like literary plane wreckage.

Then just as I had given up hope, for a fraction of a second, he paused. A chance to speak! But due to the PD I hesitated as I searched for the words that had been at ready. They were gone. My opportunity evaporated, as he renewed his rambling about various topics.

I wondered where the shut-off valve could be. I imagined another possibility - a string was slowly retracting into the back of his neck. Surely it would hit the end soon. Then, while he pulls the sting again, I would have my opening.

On one occasion, I released a grammatical salvo of my own to see if he would yield. Nope. In fact, he increased the number of words per second. I continued my volley of verbiage, but he met each word syllable for syllable. Letters flew in all directions like water from a garden hose meeting an opposing stream of comparative force. Jots, tittles and a variety of punctuation marks stuck all over our faces. Nouns, verbs, adjectives, adverbs, articles and particles covered the ceiling, walls and even our clothing.

I considered telepathy, but that meant having my thoughts under control. They usually run off like gophers and dive into their hiding places when I look in their direction, especially when I need them most. The idea of prayer entered my mind, but what means would God use to silence him concerned me. I might be sitting too close and be rendered mute myself. So, I sat there nodding at appropriate times hoping for a respite.

As the "deluge-inal" talker continued without a break, a friend walked up, looked at the oratorical debris and said, "Looks like you haven't been able to get a word in edgewise."

While fragments of diction drizzled down, I replied, "I tried laying the words flat like one would slide a piece of mail under someone's door, but that didn't work so I attempted to insert my words edgewise through crannies in the conversation, but alas no crack in the wall of words opened large enough to slip anything through. So, in answer to your comment; no, I couldn't get anything in edgewise or otherwise."

Meanwhile, the sounds emitting from the source of the verbosity continued on regardless of a new and separate conversation taking place. It seems once he got started, he became oblivious to others, or was unable to stop without drastic measures.

Suddenly, he became aware of the newcomer and stopped. My friend said, "My but you are rather verbose today."

And the talkative one said, "I know. I have been trying to loose weight, but…." And off he went down a trail of dieting woes.

The question in my mind is: who was really the one

conversationally challenged? The one with PD that loses his thoughts or words, or the one with a faulty shut off valve.

Maximum "Insultation"

I learned about minimal "insultation," in a purely unintentional manner, that one can inadvertently, and without malicious intent, insult someone. One day, after Katie had finished her usual primping period, she asked, "How does my hair look?"

I looked up from my Lazy-boy and said, "Decent. It looks decent."

She said, "Thanks a lot!" and returned to the bathroom in a miffed state of mind.

I, a man of reasonable intellect, and years of marital experience, sensed that something was amiss and amuck. I asked, "What's wrong with 'decent'?"

"It's not any better than 'fine'."

"Sure it is." Although, I thought to myself, that I never really understood what was wrong with "fine."

"When have you ever used the word 'decent'? She asked, "You don't even say 'decent.'"

"Yes, I do. 'That is a decent looking car.' See?"

"Are you comparing me to a car?"

"No. Now, you are "pretzelizing" my words. I simply mean that it is a good word to describe nice things and your hair looks nice," I said, with great care and extreme deliberation, used my tongue to remove the word "fine" from the tip of it. Yet, I sensed that I was in conversational quicksand. The more I struggled with my "decent" defense, the deeper in I wriggled. I felt the stuff restricting my movements. Then, I found myself up to my nose in trouble, and my mouth stifled - which, at first, seemed like a dire situation to be in, but the reality was, that if I couldn't reply, I couldn't cause myself further marital disharmony.

Katie added, "I texted my friend and she said that decent means "barely adequate." At that point, I realized that I had lost. I had inadvertently insulted my wife and had to place "decent" next to "fine" on the shelf of words never to be used in the context of wifely compliments. And I had inflicted minimal "insultation."

Moderate "insultation" comes as a cleverly timed and placed comeback, which I enjoy, but I am not a fan of being a recipient of insults, especially the intentional kind. Although, some are given under the guise of humor, very few people can be Don Rickles.

Past onslaughts have bruised my self-esteem, destroyed my self-confidence and consequently injured my psyche. I have discovered, in a rude and injurious manner, insults strewn about like mines in the landscape of life. As I happily trekked along, suddenly, out of the blue, I stepped squarely on a verbal explosive, which caused great injury – far beyond some stinging little slur.

I wondered where such sharpen their tongues, when, one day, I stumbled upon the training ground for these merciless inflictors of scorn – entire websites dedicated to nothing more than clever "insultation." This, no doubt, has given rise to a new subculture of people: "insulteers!" These are the musketeers of verbal swordplay and come under the heading of moderate "insultation."

Recently, I heard my doctor speak at the local Parkinson support group meeting. During his oration he used the word "insult" regarding brain trauma, specifically Parkinson's disease. Wow! It's a pretty serious insult that can cause brain damage! I found myself trying to remember an especially painful affront, but realized that replaying spiteful utterances might add insult to injury or should that be insult to insult. Hmmm, my brain began hurting, so I stopped thinking about it, just in case.

I realize that an insult can hurt, but cause traumatic effects upon my gray matter, much less reach the basil ganglia? I theorized that this is caused by attempts to allow the insult to go in one ear and out the other. However, things can go wrong, which would cause it to lodge somewhere. The only possible recourse is some evasive maneuvering by plugging both ears before the offensive statement hits or at least turning the good ear away from it. After all, if an insult was emitted, but not received, was it really an insult? The downside, though, is that the "insulteer" could be encouraged to turn up the volume, and no amount of explanation about attempting to protect oneself from brain damage would help. In fact, additional insults could be fired off in response.

I know a man that had to undergo brain surgery because all indications pointed to a brain tumor. It turned out the mass was merely scar tissue, no doubt from brain "insultation." Evidently, he had failed to wear his protective gear, or engage in evasive maneuvers, choosing instead, to endure the barrage as a ploy to tire the "insulteer" - a strategy, although not always a wise one, employed by boxers.

Since the only insults I had ever known were verbal, I looked up the word "insult" to prove the doctor wrong in his usage of "insults". Wouldn't ya know it? He was right. I didn't know what I was talking about. Oops; did I just insult myself? Is self-inflicted "insultation" possible? Hmmm.

After I thought about it though, no matter the source or intention, insults do cause damage, render someone ineffective, and can last a lifetime. So, that would make Parkinson's disease a maximum "insultation."

My "Ambitionary"

My "ambitionary" woke me up this morning. The clock said 2:17 A.M., not the time for ambition, so I tried to ignore him, but he persisted. I laid there with my mind going on fast forward like it used to before PD. Part of me wanted to get up and write, which requires all eight cylinders to do so, and they were firing, while the other reminded me of an upcoming difficult day if I did so. I thought of projects that I had put off until I felt strong enough to do it – honey-do stuff and other fixit jobs. I even thought of some new "oughta-do" tasks. My "ambitionary" even inspired me to dream of possibilities, such as starting some new ministry. With much determination, I stayed in bed putting off my "ambitionary" until daylight. I fell asleep again and woke up at the normal time with the usual PD stiffness and soreness. What happened to my "ambitionary?" Argh, he didn't wait until I got up for the day! I was so looking forward to a day of productivity.

I begin my days by taking my meds and hoping they will bring normalcy, but that is unpredictable, unreliable and not guaranteed, so I didn't get my hopes up. Days later, (I am not sure how long) I set out pushing myself along like most days, when my "ambitionary" made a surprise visit in the morning. My mind cleared. I went through my morning stretches, a bit of stationary bike riding, and my daily devotional. I then started on the list. My "ambitionary" came up with ideas of things to do, but I already had too much to do – they had been put off until a day like this. I worked on a sermon and chased rabbits until I grew tired of it and had to finish the message at hand. Since I used to have boundless energy, my "ambitionary" expected me to be able to spend time working on various projects non-stop until bedtime. Then just as quickly as he came, he was gone and it was only mid afternoon. I used to be able to keep up with him, but that guy has too much energy nowadays.

The down side is that after a good day with my "ambitionary" I always pay for our escapades. Sure enough, the next few days I had more stiffness, soreness and fatigue, and my mind turned to oatmeal. My bed became a good comforter until I recovered. Sometimes the downtime may last for a couple of weeks. I vowed I would behave myself the next time my "ambitionary" shows up, but he will probably hoodwink me again.

"Paddletales"

The idea of pedaling as a benefit to "PWP's" has been getting more popular lately. One day while at Lake Alvin, a nearby lake, my wife and I noticed a family in a paddleboat. We decided that would be a nice way to spend quality time together. Besides, the paddling is actually pedaling which runs a paddle beneath the boat, so pedaling a paddle ought to be a good thing.

The very next Sunday, I made a run to the local grocery store for frappuccinos and noticed a white and blue paddleboat sitting outside the entrance next to a porch swing. "Why would a grocery store have a paddleboat?" I asked myself.

"To sell, I suppose." I said to me as I walked inside.

Then, I suggested to myself, "Why don't you ask someone about it?"

So, I took my advice and asked a clerk. A pained expression came over the young lady's face, as if an old guy had asked her something totally nonsensical and said, "A what?"

"A paddleboat, could you ask a manager?" I asked, attempting to encourage the clerk to show some initiative.

"Ok." She semi-cheerfully responded and started to walk away, turned back and asked. "You want to know about what again?"

"A paddleboat." I re-informed her.

"A paddleboat? A paddleboat." She repeated to herself as if she had never heard of such a thing.

"Yup. It is outside the front door on the sidewalk." I enlightened her because she just might peak outside the door to see the mysterious item.

"Ok." and off she went and returned momentarily with a manager. They were conversing as they approached. I imagined her saying something like, "There's, like, this ol' guy up front, and like, he would be quite handsome if he was younger, but seemed confused, or something, and um, would you, um, talk to him? He wants to know something about a paddle-something, or something." The manager had a look of befuddlement as he greeted me.

"I was wondering what the story is on the paddleboat outside the front door." I said attempting to cover all potential questions.

"Paddleboat?" He looked puzzled, probably trying to decipher the clerk's info and merging it with my request in his mind. Just when I was losing hope, his eyes displayed recognition as he said slowly. "Oh! You…mean…the…paddle…boat!"

"Yup. That would be it." I responded. "What is the story on it?"

"We sold it." He said, as if that ended the discussion.

"I see." I felt disappointed, yet continued on despite his disheartening announcement. "Do you know if the other stores have any?"

"No, I don't." He replied, probably hoping that this middle-aged nuisance would go away.

My curiosity welled up inside, looking for release. So, rather than have it ooze out my ears and leave a mess on the floor, I asked; "How did your grocery stores end up with paddleboats anyway?"

"Well, each store received one from some company as a reward for good sales." He explained, but was unsure which company did so.

I went home and called the other stores in town. A store way on the other side of town had one left, and they promised that the manager, privy to such information, would get back with me. He called back in the afternoon and said they would let it go for half price. So, I bought it.

We had now joined the elite group of people that could say they go boating on the weekends. I looked forward to letting Katie know that we could heartily sing nautical songs like the Gilligan's Island theme song, but we would only do so when our grown kids are with us in the middle of the lake for optimum effect. Few things compare with giving ones grown children no escape while embarrassing them; although, one can end up covered in lake water, if not careful because as adults they do not fear parental repercussions.

Next, we needed to secure flotation devices (AKA life jackets) to be legal and to be prepared in case our world turned upside down on the lake. We even found one for our Yorkie. It strapped around him securely, and a suitcase style handle sprouted from the top for easy handling. We were ready.

The next available day, we packed a picnic lunch, loaded the paddleboat on the pickup, strapped it down tightly and headed for a nearby "no wake" lake. Only slow moving boats and such were allowed, so we fit in. Young speed-loving men, such as my son, feel that a whole lot of pedaling occurs without much of an acceleration benefit, but then, the oxymoronic idea of high speed in a paddleboat is fraught with danger.

We unloaded the boat and set it in the water. "Have you changed the rudder to the non-shipping position?" Katie asked.

"I looked at it and it looked fine to me." I replied.

"Are you sure? It has a sticker with a picture explaining it." She quizzed me further.

"I looked at it and it looks fine to me." I insisted.

"OK, if you say so, but..." She warned as we put the boat in the water.

Climbing in the boat proved to be exciting because the boat attempted evasive maneuvers when weight pressed down on it. It moved down and away from whoever stepped in it. Shrieking and splashing sounds motivated me to hold the boat in place as Katie and Dickens got in. I then climbed on board from the dock side, but the boat tried to scoot out from under my foot and caused more shrieking and splashing sounds. The good news is that we found ourselves sitting in the front pedal pusher seats with minimal wetness.

Our maiden voyage proved uneventful and relaxing other than having to unify our pedaling. If one pedals and the other doesn't, the pedals smack, strike and stimulate much movement from the non-pedaler. I discovered that increasing the speed at such a time is not good for one's well-being either. Katie had no problem resorting to physicality by smacking my arm in order to end bruise infliction upon her shins. Thus, unified pedaling is the preferable method.

Once we polished our technique (in other words, I behaved myself) the paddling went well; although, the steering didn't seem very responsive. It took a lot of verbal assistance on my part to get it to obey the turning of the rudder. We got a good workout when we bucked the wind and enjoyed drifting along with it on the return voyage. We loved listening to the birds sing, and seeing an occasional carp jump. The deciduous foliage covering the hilly slopes down to the water added to the pleasantry. We enjoyed our outing. Dickens did, too, once he had something soft to sit on – which after a while, we sympathized with him, because the hard plastic seats grew harder through the day.

As we loaded the boat on the pickup to head home, I noticed something. "Katie, look at this. The rudder is still in the shipping position. No wonder it didn't respond well," I stated, as if I had discovered something profound.

"Let me remind you, that I reminded you to check it before we put it in the water." She gleefully pointed out.

"I suppose I should have actually read the instructions closer - well okay, read them in the first place." I admitted.

I heard a sigh and looked in Katie's direction and noted her "gloatation" device had been activated. "Could you help me, please?" I said, obviously acknowledging that she was right.

Our next boating trip went smoothly, except that we forgot to bring towels, but, since water evaporates, we didn't worry about it. Dickens missed his soft bedding made of towels, so he restlessly wandered about the boat. Since the wind was blowing in a different direction than our last outing, we were able to explore the other end of the lake. As we drifted along with the wind, Dickens decided to check out the water from the right rear passenger seat. He leaned over, looked back at me as if to say, "This is the biggest puddle I have ever seen!" and stepped off the boat.

He did not hit bottom as he expected, but ended up engaging in some paddling of his own. Since he had never previously experienced the world going out from under him, this alien environment disoriented and confused him. However, after he bobbed to the surface with the assistance of his canine lifejacket, dogpaddle instinct automatically engaged. We reversed the paddling procedure to intercept him and called to him because he was going full speed, but without a definite destination in mind. Finally, he realized the voices he heard were familiar and began swimming for the boat. The handle on his floatation device came in very handy for Katie to pick him up out of the lake. The water dripping off him filled the seating area on the right side of the boat, prompting Katie to mention, in a resolute manner, that we should have had some towels. The reminder that water evaporates did little to change her mindset. Towels have now moved to the top of the list to bring on next boating adventure. Dickens' Yorkie-do was totally ruined and he didn't seem to enjoy the trip as much as a soggy doggie, yet there were times he looked as if he would try DIY paddling again.

Although at times, Katie out-pedaled me, the "tandemness" helped my pace and endorphin levels and we couldn't beat the quality time. Certainly, there will be more "paddletales" in store, so stay tuned.

I Am My Own Doppelganger

All my life I have experienced a strange phenomenon that afflicts only me and no one else in my family. My stuff disappears. That's right. I know without a doubt where I left the item in question and when I go to retrieve it – it's gone! Obviously, somebody takes it. That is the only explanation. However, no one in the family ever 'fesses up. In fact, they smirk and question my theory as if I said something far-fetched in an effort to cover my own foibles. Through my years of going hither and yon in this world I have learned that I have a doppelganger – he is the culprit.

A doppelganger is the ghost or apparition of a living person. "Doppel" means double while "ganger" comes from "gang" with this definition: "a set of like tools, machines, components, etc., designed or arranged to work together"[3] My clone would be a real live copy of me, my reflection a real time likeness of me, and my shadow is merely a mime of me. So, my doppelganger is my ghostly me that is supposed to work with me as part of a team but, instead, opts for impish behavior.

I cannot see my doppelganger due to his invisibility, however I see evidence of his existence quite often, especially now that I am stranded on the ledge near the top of the hill (50+ is *not* over the hill). He definitely has redoubled his efforts to drive me nuts once PD came along by hiding more of my things than ever.

---

[3] Webster's New World Dictionary & Thesaurus, Accent Software International, Macmillan Publishers, Version 2.0, 1998, "gang" definition #2.

I related my doppelganger discovery to my wife, after another episode of missing glasses. She showed her support by saying I was the one losing it in more ways than one. She claims I put items in strange places myself and that nobody is hiding my stuff. Her wild accusations have roughed up my self-esteem considerably.

The other day she asked me to get some newspapers that she had forgotten in the car. I looked inside the front seat area, got out, closed the door, then opened the back door and looked in the backseat area – nothing but black upholstery and carpet. I informed her that the papers were definitely NOT in the car. She asked if she needed to go look. I told her to go ahead. After approximately forty-seven seconds, she walked back in the house with the newspapers and said that I can't find anything unless it falls into my outstretched hands. Frustration and embarrassment set in, causing mumbling and grumbling. The fact is the newspapers weren't there when I looked for them. My doppelganger hid them from me. Worst of all, he put them back before she found them in the very same place I had just thoroughly searched.

My doppelganger is out to drive me crazy. I sat down to work on a crossword puzzle the other day, and he had filled in some of the blanks – in my handwriting. Not only that, but some were wrong! One time I packed my lunch for work; but on lunch break I discovered that it wasn't in my lunchbox – my doppelganger had taken it out and put it on the counter for Katie to find later.

Another time I took a bowl and juice glass out of the cupboard and placed them on the counter for my breakfast.

While I filled the bowl with cereal and the glass with juice, he took out the same things and put them on the table before I got there!

He also likes to rearrange my shoes in the closet so that I wear my slippers to church instead of my dress shoes. When that happens I praise God that they are not fuzzy pink bunny slippers!

Today, I received a call from our church secretary. She had difficulty speaking because her ha-ha's and tee-hee's got tangled up in the syllables. It seems the employees at the county jail reported they had received an envelope containing some amusement from my church. It held a blank form requesting chaplaincy clearance, and since they already had lots of those, they figured somebody blundered seriously. She struggled to breathe between her chuckles and chortles as she explained that she had called various members to identify the possible blunderbuss. Evidently this proved very entertaining for her and them. It turns out that my doppelganger had stuffed it in an envelope before I could fill it out and mailed it. I am sure he enjoyed the jocularity, as well.

Sometimes I wonder about my doppelganger. Does he have a name? Perhaps he is really Frank my fictitious man Friday. No, Frank is the one who doesn't do things. Whenever something I was supposed to do has gone undone, Frank, who is the epitome of undependability, gets the blame. Katie understands this concept. She says that Frances, her imaginary maid is the same way. I have tried to explain to Katie that, although my doppelganger is invisible, he is real (unlike Frank) and is the one who pulls pranks on me. I'm not sure whether she was mocking when she suggested his name is Nivek, sort of a mirror image of Kevin (niveK|Kevin).

Recently, I planned a meeting with my doppelganger to discuss his behavior. I even bribed him with cookies and hot chocolate. But then I discovered the cookies I absolutely positively knew were in the cupboard had disappeared. I dutifully told Katie that somebody had stolen my cookies. She looked at me with disbelief splashed all over her face - or maybe it was soapy water - and said that it must have been Nivek, my doppelganger.

She believes!

Cerebral Freezer Burn

I am no expert. I know a little bit about everything and a lot of nothing, and since the experts do not seem to know with absolute certainty what causes PD, I feel I can relate my theory. Some say it is hereditary, some say it is not. Some say it is caused by chemicals, others by heavy metals, and some have even called it an auto-immune disorder. But, this morning, an idea that I believe could seriously change the direction of research hit me in the forehead while quickly downing my morning class of COLD orange juice. At first my brain occupied itself with pain stoppage, then, after the intensity subsided, I wondered if I had sustained any brain damage. After the slushiness in my mind melted, thinking set in.

I began letting my mind wander – not far because it may wander out on the street, get hit by a car or it could simply vanish. For example, one time while at work, I told my boss that I had lost my mind and asked him if he had seen it. He said he had stepped in something back yonder, and maybe that was it. After close examination, the gooey substance turned out to be gum, which eased my anxiety, and as quietly as it wandered off, my mind came back to me.

Since my brain felt like it had experienced trauma from my cold juice (that which kids commonly refer to as an ice cream headache AKA an ICHA) – I realized it could very possibly cause brain damage. The boys that I remember consuming frozen deserts to intentionally, and with premeditation, give themselves brain freezes seemed a little off center, but then again, maybe they gave themselves

ICHA's because they were already a little off. I'm getting dizzy just trying to reason that one out.

Businesses have gone crazy with warning labels and disclaimers on their products. People have sued over their coffee being hot, and burning them because they carelessly spilled it upon their person. Thusly, it seems it would behoove manufacturers to put a warning label similar to this on frozen deserts: "WARNING: gulping this product down in a rapid and reckless manner could lead to temporary frontal lobe pain. Repeated abuse of this frozen product could lead to permanent cerebral freezer burn."

The problem with young boys and warnings is that boys must test the truthfulness of said caution. "Hey, I have an idea, let's see who can eat this ice cream sundae fastest," says the leader of the pack.

"But the warning label says it could cause a temporary headache," warns the conscience of the group.

"COOL, let's do it and see who is the toughest!" cheers the group in unison and they gulp down the frozen desert until grimacing faces and strange groaning sounds occur.

"Guys, we can't do that very often, or we could get cerebral freezer burn," the conscience speaks up again. "It says so on the label."

"Really? Let's do it again," and they do, while laughing at each other's funny faces. If only we could fast forward fifty years, and see how many are dealing with the consequences of self-induced brain-freezes.

I truly believe I am onto something here. My theory is that ICHA's cause PD. Since boys willingly self-induce themselves with brain-freezing, it naturally follows the parameters of logic that Parkinson's is more prevalent in guys. A popular idea is that Parkinson's disease came along with the chemicals associated with industrialization. However, along with said industrialization came refrigeration, and thus ice cream and frozen deserts. The validity to this concept cannot be argued because no research on ICHA's has been conducted. Therefore, the repercussions of freezing one's brain temporarily, yet frequently, are unknown. In like manner, no one has looked for an association between PD and cerebral freezer burn – until me.

Maybe this phenomenon will be named after me, and I can have my very own flower as a symbol (like the tulip for PD), perhaps a mottled variety of daffodil called the "Boekhoffian" daffodil.

Bonus Material

I would like to make you an offer that is easy to refuse. I would like to give away my Early Onset Parkinson's disease. I have found that my slow moving nicely equipped model could give someone endearing complications to their life. This version comes with the basic bradykinesia, rigidity and postural issues, which currently respond to the meds readily. The predominant option of rigidity will challenge you with stiffness and soreness during off times. I recommend a daily regimen of stretching and exercise to properly care for it and prevent voiding the bogus warranty. At very quiet times, you can also exercise to the sound of the cogwheel effect in the left arm. Plus the times of sleeplessness and emotional upheavals will give your life variety.

Its deceptively degenerating nature could lend to some future surprises not apparent today (besides the depreciation in value of your functionality). If you choose to acquire my version of PD, with its uncharted future, you may one day experience "freezing" (despite the warm temperature), facial masking (a plasticized version of your own face), soft muffled speech, a tendency to fall backwards, or walk like Tim Conway's old man (short shuffling steps). You might have difficulty blinking (which aids in avoiding misunderstandings from winking) and swallowing (you won't swallow those tall tales shared by your buddies) as well as constipation, and oily skin (saves money on hand lotion). Of course, the most thrilling of all would be dementia, but I forget what that is.

I also have a couple of bonus features not included in the basic package. The first and most worthy of mentioning is my myoclonus. It is a left-sided muscle jerk that varies in intensity and location. Consequently, my wife isn't the only one to wake up with a jerk. The advantage is that the jerkiness can be a great conversation piece when others notice it, especially knocking over a beverage at a restaurant.

The second is Essential Tremor. Since it isn't in the usual PD package I wondered why it is essential and would have opted out if I could. It doesn't usually show itself except in times of stress or occasionally during off times. Thus, I am willing to throw it in with the deal.

Some other extras are active muscles which twitch in a low-key manner, buzzing spots, and an occasional Charley Horse. A lousy sense of smell contributes to the neutrality of life. This is an advantage in stinky situations, but a disadvantage when one wants to enjoy the wonderful fragrances of a bakery.

There is no money down, but you will pay the rest of your life for acquiring PD. Just think of the negativity you can undergo while missing out on other things. So, don't act now and you may miss out on the experience of a lifetime![4]

---

[4] If you would like more information on PD contact: National Parkinson Foundation South Dakota Chapter, 1000 N West Ave, Suite 220, Sioux Falls, SD 57104, 605-271-6113, www.npfsouthdakota.org. Email: info@parkinsonsd.org.

The Problem That Never Was

I had a problem with someone who had a problem the other day. The problem was, they really didn't have a problem, and that was their problem. They simply wanted to have a problem, so they manufactured a problem and then embarked on problem promotion by presenting it to me as my problem. Now, I had a problem. How does one fix a problem that never was? That in itself poses a problem.

The real problem for me was not the pseudo-problem itself, but that the problem promotion caused stress, and stress causes problems with my PD. At problematic times like these, I can experience jerking and twitching, my tremor comes out to play and my myoclonus joins the physical anarchy. I don't normally have a problem with such a muscular free-for-all, unless they are "problematized" by a problem. Plus, the severity of the symptoms displays the severity of the problem.

The problem also exposed a problem I hadn't realized I had a problem with – anxiety (something PWP's know well, I am told). Thus, the problem-that-never-was caused a problem concerning the angst associated with potential problems. There is nothing like anxiety to intensify, exacerbate and otherwise heighten one's awareness of the miniscule. What is normally considered a non-issue is magnified through the lens of anxiety and becomes an enhanced problem. Plus, anxiety can create new problems-that-never-were, relating to the original problem-that-never-was.

Problems have always been a problem for me, but now

with my PD the problems cause more problems, which enhance other problems. The more I want my "problematized" body to calm, the greater the problem becomes through anxiety. The problem is removing the problem that caused my problem to become a problem. Once that problem is gone the other problems dissipate, as well.

My request is a preemptive strike against problems: if my problem is due to your problem, and if you really don't have a problem, then please don't create a problem-that-never-was and we will be problem-free, stress free and anxiety free, thank you!

My Pocket Watch

All my life I have entertained the notion of a pocket watch. I imagined my distinguished self pulling out my gold time piece from my pocket, matching chain glittering, as I open the engraved cover reciting the time to myself. However, I never discovered a Timex pocket watch, so the majority of my life I ended up with the popular wristwatch.

The main problem with wristwatches is they must be strapped to my forearm. It is a most annoying process to balance the watch on my arm, press it against my leg to steady the strap. Then, attempt to thread the other strap through the clasp and put the little pointy thing through the appropriate hole, followed by pushing the strap through the other side of the clasp. This is irritating enough without Parkinson's but reaches the exasperation point on bad days when my hands hurt badly or shake.

The other choice available was the chrome expandable stretchable twist-a-flex style band. This alleviated the previous problem, but I discovered it grabbed arm hair and pulled on the hairs slowly and persistently until the area had become bald. On one occasion I scratched my nose and lowered my hand quickly only to have the band grab some mustache whiskers. Good night! I thought a piece of my lip had been torn away. I looked at the watchband, just a few whiskers. I looked in the mirror, but no noticeable damage other than my eyes still tearing and my lip complaining about the violence inflicted upon it.

Another disadvantage is the wristwatch wearer's tan.

As the arm tans through the summer, the skin under the watch stays cave-dweller white. Not much of a problem unless one forgets to put on the watch or loses it. Then the white strip flashes loudly to passersby that my memory failed me or some terrible fate had happened to my time piece.

My family quit buying me watches as gifts because of another difficulty I experienced with watches; I would accidentally scrape them against things. This left scratches across the crystal. I tried spinning the face to the inside of my forearm, but this annoyed my wrist to such a degree I had to remove the watch. Sometimes, unbeknownst to me, the strap would release its grip and slip off my arm. I would discover it later when I went to check the time and a white band of skin smiled at me.

I went through watches constantly, so I never invested much money in them. I had some that looked really cool, some that kept track of the date and time, some that noted military time, some that looked like a compass, some gold, some silver, some stainless steal, some black plastic, some digital and some analog – never had a Mickey Mouse one though.

Guess what? I have found the pocket watch of my most vivid imaginings. I no longer have to battle with a clasp on the band or worry about it yanking out my mustache. It is a digital pocket watch – who'd a thunk it? I can set several alarms so I never forget to take my meds at the correct times, which is very important to have good days. What a blessing! Instead of making an obnoxious jangling sound it can play a tune. I just can't get used to trying to figure out whether it is the store's atmospheric music or my pocket watch, so I left the old style ring setting alone. Better than that, I can also turn off the ring and have it vibrate when it alarms. Sometimes though, when it gets between my wallet and my leg and then goes off my mind says I am being electrocuted and I reflexively jump. This, in turn, brings surprised reactions from people around me especially if I holler. Knowing their concern, I remove my pocket watch from my pocket, show it to them and explain that it is just my pocket watch alarm going off, nothing to worry about. I then nonchalantly open the cover, shut it off and put it in back in my pocket.

My pocket watch constantly apprises me the day and date, as well as the time. I can even change it to read military time. I can vary the background of the face by choosing one of several provided photographic choices. Technology has advanced the pocket watch to the point that I can send messages to people with it. I can talk to anyone I want by just dialing their phone number on the keypad, almost like Captain Kirk's communicator. This pocket watch has something called speed dial. Just press one number and I can talk to somebody.

My new pocket watch also takes pictures of stuff. The downside of this gizmo is that it has a mind of its own and sometimes takes pictures of the inside of my pocket leaving me with several pictures of blackness stored in it.

I discovered that I have the choice of a stopwatch as well! I can time myself doing various activities or, better yet, time others. However, this is the most dangerous of all the options. A word of caution: never use this selection as a motivational device to encourage greater speed out of your wife.

I can record future appointments on the calendar and it will remind me prior to the engagement with a chime, tune or obnoxious sound, if I choose to record one into it. On that notation, I can record myself telling myself to do something or I will have to answer to me later. What a timepiece!

I figured out another feature in the darkest of night. It can work as a flashlight, howbeit a dim one. This luminous option has saved me on several occasions from crashing into furniture on my midnight treks to the latrine.

I am told I can purchase a "nagivator" service, which can tell me where to turn and so forth in a nagging fashion; hence the name I suppose. Who could have imagined pocket watches could be a compass, too! Sorry Dick Tracy, but this beats your TV wristwatch.

I understand that I can get Bluetooth. Why would anyone want a blue tooth? Perhaps to color coordinate with "smurf" colored hair, I suppose. I have also been informed that I can have games installed on it to help pass the time – all these features, and more for small additional monthly fees, of course.

What a wonderful pocket watch! Shazam, what will they think of next?

Disaster Assistance

Allowing me to do something in the kitchen has always been a decision somewhere between bravery and foolhardiness according to my wife and kids. They consider an imminent disaster as fact. My Parkinson's disease has also contributed to the phenomenon my family calls the "cascade effect," which they use exclusively pertaining to my messes. Let me explain.

Since we have become empty-nesters and I lost my job due to a back injury and PD, I have endeavored to contribute in the domestic duties department. Thus, I usually just warm up some leftovers and have them ready to serve the moment my wife gets in the door from her job.

One day, I decided to make pancakes and link sausages for our noon meal. I proceeded to take out the small box of frozen sausages and put them in a frying pan with a little water to cook. I then secured the box of Bisquick from the cabinet, spent a few minutes trying to find the instructions for simple pancakes (in English) measured out the powder, poured some milk and threw an egg into a bowl (without the shell, c'mon now). After a little thought, I remembered my wife had a handheld drill-like apparatus she used for mixing cookie dough. I figured that ought to work. Before long I had the Hamilton Beach electric mixer flinging the ingredients about in the stainless steel mixing bowl. Yes, success!

No, not so, the runniness of the batter indicated an error in the quantity of one of the liquids. To thicken the batter, I set out to add more Bisquick. I allowed the mixer to balance in the batter and bowl while I set out to find the Bisquick box once again. I had just barely gotten the box in hand when I heard a clunk/splat/drip-drip-drip sound. I discovered the bowl had tipped over and sloshed its runny contents down the face of the cabinets. The batter cascaded downward into the two top drawers that I had inadvertently left open a bit. Argh.

I abandoned the box and dashed over to stop the flow of ooze. At this point, I discovered the slippery puddle on the floor where our Yorkie, who normally works as a professional squeaker of dog toys, had embarked on a mission of disaster assistance by licking up as much of the mixture as he could. After slowing the flow by throwing towels on the counter, I discovered that the top drawer had received a large amount squarely in the silverware tray. The next drawer down had no tray, but held a bunch of utensils and other miscellaneous kitchen aides now embedded in pancake batter. The cascade effect had held true – literally.

Meanwhile back on the stove, the sausages started turning into carbon, causing a smelly haze to waft throughout the house. I noticed it before the smoke alarm did, took the frying pan off the burner, set it outside and opened all the windows.

I felt I had things under control, until I looked at our Yorkie, T-Bone Dickens, as he slid by me smearing his body along the floor as if he had just received a bath. Evidently, Dickens had placed himself strategically underfoot hoping for morsels from the project or else he had sensed a flood of savoriness coming his way. The matted crusty look of his coat indicated that he had been at the epicenter and then had begun spreading goo throughout the living room and dining room carpet. Due to my preoccupation with the batter inundation in the kitchen, some time had elapsed; consequently, I discovered that if you allow pancake batter to dry, it will vacuum out of the carpet pretty well.

In order to minimize the mess before my wife's imminent arrival, I set out to clean it up. I wiped out drawers and the cabinet, mopped the floor, washed dishes, and hoped the smoke smell had dissipated satisfactorily.

I had just finished shampooing and blow drying Dickens as my wife arrived. I met her at the car and explained the absence of pancakes and the reason for the smoky odor. I also had to disclose that Dickens didn't really have dandruff; I simply hadn't gotten all the batter out of his hair. I also related to her that Dickens had worked in disaster assistance, not disaster relief mind you, but had, in fact, assisted with the magnitude of said disaster.

And now, a word from the pastor that resides within me[5]

---

[5] Even though the tone of this essay is different than those previous, I have included it because the motivation in writing it was the same – Parkinson's disease, and, also, because I want to help others. Besides, the pastor in me wanted a chance to speak, as well.

My Uninvited Guest

Some of us will experience the arrival of an uninvited and unwanted guest sometime in our lives. I am talking about a life changing illness or physical handicap due to an accident. Some may even hear the word "terminal" regarding their uninvited guest.

Mine turned out to be Parkinson's disease. For years I didn't know what was happening to me. For lack of a name I called it UG (short for Univited Guest). It sounded like "ugh", which described how I felt much of the time. I knew UG was here to stay before the neurologist told me the news. I simply wanted a name to know how to deal with UG and to give my symptoms credibility. I knew that I was not a hypochondriac, that it was not a vitamin deficiency, that it wasn't due to the aspartame in diet pop (which I didn't drink), and that it wasn't allergies, or depression. I struggled with coming to terms with it – especially the unknown.

When an uninvited guest arrives, what can we do? How do we find the peace of God in the midst of such a life-altering event? First of all, before God can help us, there must be a foundation. We must have a relationship with Him. If we have not trusted Christ as our Savior, then we are on the wrong side of a relationship with Him. We are unforgiven, unrighteous - an enemy of His. However, that can be changed. The uninvited guest that has moved into our lives may be our catalyst to seek God.

The Bible says that we must trust Christ as our Savior to ensure the fact that we will spend our eternity in heaven.

Our eternal life begins at the day of salvation. The day we get saved is the day our life changes. The Holy Spirit lives within us and <u>nothing</u> will be the same. On that day, God becomes our personal God, Jesus becomes our personal Savior, and the Holy Spirit becomes our personal Counselor. He now guides and directs our life. He fills us with hope, peace, love and joy. He now gives us a reason to live, forgiveness of sins, a sure hope of heaven, and peace that passes understanding. Everyone can have this wonderful relationship with Jesus. If we are to benefit from the promises and truths contained in the rest of this essay, we must have Christ as our Savior.

The promise: *1 John 5:13 These things have I written unto you that believe on the name of the Son of God; that **ye may know that ye have eternal life**, and that ye may believe on the name of the Son of God.*

All have sinned: *Romans 3:23 For all have sinned, and come short of the glory of God.* Which leaves us in a bad state *John 3:18 He that believeth on him is not condemned: but he that believeth not is condemned already, because he hath not believed in the name of the only begotten Son of God.*

Sin's penalty: *Romans 6:23 For the wages of sin is death; but the gift of God is eternal life through Jesus Christ our Lord.*

Sin's Penalty must be paid: *Hebrews 9:22 And almost all things are by the law purged with blood; and without shedding of blood is no remission.*

Sin's Penalty Was Paid: *Romans 5:8 But God commendeth his love toward us, in that, while we were yet sinners, Christ died for us. 1 Corinthians 15:3 For I delivered unto you first of all that which I also received, how that Christ died for our sins according to the scriptures.*

You must repent: *Isaiah 55:7 Let the wicked forsake his way, and the unrighteous man his thoughts: and let him return unto the LORD, and he will have mercy upon him; and to our God, for he will abundantly pardon.*

You must receive Christ: *Acts 4:12 Neither is there salvation in any other: for there is none other name under heaven given among men, whereby we must be saved. John 14:6 Jesus saith unto him, I am the way, the truth, and the life: no man cometh unto the Father, but by me.*

You can be saved today: *Romans 10:9, 13 That if thou shalt confess with thy mouth the Lord Jesus, and shalt believe in thine heart that God hath raised him from the dead, thou shalt be saved. For whosoever shall call upon the name of the Lord shall be saved.*

What we must do:

* Admit our need (I am a condemned sinner).

* Be willing to turn from our sin (repent).

* Believe that Jesus Christ died for us on the cross.

* Through prayer, ask God to save us through the death, burial and resurrection of Jesus.

At this point Jesus becomes our Master *1 Corinthians*

6:19-20 What? know ye not that your body is the temple of the Holy Ghost which is in you, which ye have of God, and ye are not your own? For ye are bought with a price: therefore glorify God in your body, and in your spirit, which are God's. Our former unloving cruel master was the devil. We now have a loving Master that cares for us and provides for us as long as we put Him first—the place a master should have in a servant's life. *Matthew 6:33 But seek ye first the kingdom of God, and his righteousness; and all these things shall be added unto you.*

Even though we have a relationship with God, we may have a difficult time understanding Him. Many have been misled to believe that God will always heal. Certainly God can heal if He wishes to do so, but He does not always heal. He may have other plans. Paul asked God to heal him, but God did not. Instead, He promised to be with him through the ordeal *2 Corinthians 12:7-9 And lest I should be exalted above measure through the abundance of the revelations, there was given to me a thorn in the flesh, the messenger of Satan to buffet me, lest I should be exalted above measure. For this thing I besought the Lord thrice, that it might depart from me. And he said unto me, my grace is sufficient for thee: for my strength is made perfect in weakness. Most gladly therefore will I rather glory in my infirmities, that the power of Christ may rest upon me. Therefore I take pleasure in infirmities, in reproaches, in necessities, in persecutions, in distresses for Christ's sake: for when I am weak, then am I strong.* Notice how Paul's attitude changed when he realized that God could use him better because he had an uninvited guest. He gloried in his infirmity. As you read the verse, try taking "infirmity" out and replacing it with PD, or whatever your UG may be.

Jesus even had the same attitude when it came to the cross. *Matthew 26:39 And he went a little farther, and fell on his face, and prayed, saying, O my Father, if it be possible, let this cup pass from me: nevertheless not as I well, but as thou wilt.* We learn that we are to be Christ-like, so take your example from Him – to be submissive to the will of your Father.

Rest assured, God is in control of circumstances that <u>seem</u> to be out of control.

The Bible is our source of victory. It will strengthen us, renew us, help heal our broken heart, sustain us and give us answers. *Philippians 4:13 I can do all things through Christ which strengtheneth me. Psalms 119:50 This is my comfort in my affliction: for thy word hath quickened me. Psalms 119:165 Great peace have they which love thy law: and nothing shall offend them.*

Pray. We need to talk to God often. *Philippians 4:6-7 Be careful for nothing; but in every thing by prayer and supplication with thankgiving let your requests be made known unto God. And the peace of God, which passeth all understanding, shall keep your hearts and minds through Christ Jesus.* We should keep a prayer journal (like a diary) to record answers. It can become an encouragement to us to review when times are tough. It will help us to realize that God sees us through the trials to the end.

Having the right attitude can make all the difference in our life *Hebrews 13:5 Let your conversation be without covetousness; and be content with such things as ye have: for he hath said, I well never leave thee, nor forsake thee.*

Get control of our negative thoughts *2 Corinthians 10:5 Casting down imaginations, and every high thing that exalteth itself against the knowledge of God, and bringing into captivity every thought to the obedience of Christ; Ephesians 4:23 And be renewed in the spirit of your mind; 2 Timothy 1:7 For God hath not given us the spirit of fear; but of power, and of love, and of a sound mind.*

Don't require that others constantly encourage us because we are constantly down, discouraged and defeated. When we have complete trust in the Lord then we well set the tone and the attitude. People will love and respect us for it and it will glorify God. *Philippians 2:4 Look not every man on his own things, but every man also on the things of others. Acts 20:35…remember the words of the Lord Jesus, how he said, It is more blessed to give than to receive.* This helps us keep our minds occupied and gives our lives purpose.

Stay active *Colossians 3:17 And whatsoever ye do in word or deed, do all in the name of the Lord Jesus, giving thanks to God and the Father by him.* We must learn our everchanging limits, don't overdo. Do what we can in moderation. Sometimes we may overdo on the good days and be down for several days afterward. It is better to pace ourselves on the good days to ensure more good days. On the bad days we may have to force ourselves to do something. Set goals, which will help motivate on bad days. We need to go to church, we need the fellowship of other Christians. We need the preaching of God's Word. Even if we feel bad, we need to go anyway. Go other places. Spend time with your family. Enjoy the little things of life.

One of the first responses we will experience when an uninvited guest arrives is, "Why?" What frustration to have the direction of our lives changed! What is to happen now? The thing to keep in mind is that God has a purpose for our lives *2 Timothy 1:9 Who hath saved us, and called us with an holy calling, not according to our works, but according to his own purpose and grace, which was given us in Christ Jesus before the world began.* We may struggle and rebel a bit because we may not be willing to begin a new chapter in our lives, *Proverbs 16:9 A man's heart deviseth his way: but the LORD directeth his steps.* However, some understanding can help us adjust.

Here are some reasons for the uninvited guest.

To teach us to trust in His purpose *(Romans 8:28)*.

To teach us dependence on Him *(Psalms 37:23-24)*.

To teach us how to comfort others *(2 Corinthians 1:3-7)*.

To teach us that we can have joy in spite of the uninvited guest *(1 Peter 4:12- 13)*. (Remove "fiery trial" and fill in the name of your uninvited guest).

To develop maturity and bring spiritual growth in our lives *(James 1:3-5)*.

To get us into God's Word *(Psalms 119:71)*.

To keep us on the right path (*Psalms 119:67*).

To improve our prayer life (*Isaiah 26:16*).

To open new doors of witnessing *(Philippians 1:12-13)*.

To adjust our priorities (*Philippians 1:21; Psalms 90:12*).

God does not give us more than we can handle *1 Corinthinas 10:13 There hath no temptation taken us but such as is common to man: but God is faithful, who well not suffer us to be tempted above that ye are able; but will with the temptation also make a way to escape, that ye may be able to bear it.* We must trust in Him more than ever. He does not wish to make us **bitter**, but **better**. Why let our uninvited guest defeat us? We may not have a choice in our circumstances, but we have a choice in our attitude. Choose God today!

If you would like further spiritual help please contact:

Eastside Baptist Church,

6101 E 49th Street,
Sioux Falls, SD 57110

605-336-1034

website: eastsidesf.org

Glossary

Ambitionary: The personification of my ambition.

Appy: Short for appendectomy.

Basal Ganglia: The part of the brain affected by Parkinson's.

Bewilderness: The state of being lost and bewildered. A play on the word "wilderness."

Bewildebeast: A play on the word "wildebeast," meaning one in a bewildered state.

Bleepazoid: One who, or that which, must be bleeped; similar to the procedure TV utilizes when they insert a bleep sound in place of a curse word (if only one could invent a bleeper that could obliterate profanity in real time).

Boekhoffian: Named after my last name, Boekhoff. Seems conceivable doesn't it? The sound even rolls off the tongue well.

Bonehead English: The level of English classes geared for boneheads.

Bondo: Plastic autobody filler.

Buzzooka: A fictional weapon of mass insect destruction.

Cahooterize: The state of being in cahoots, or in league with another, usually applied to unsavory behavior or a conspiracy.

Cantankerosity: A cantankerous or crabby condition.

Charley Horse: Muscle cramps.

Cinderfella: A masculine version of the poor and oppressed Cinderella as she mopped and cleaned.

Clutterized: Something usedful turned into clutter.

Cobblized: Something that has been "repaired" in a crude and rude manner.

Contortium: A torture chamber in which one is forced into being a contortionist.

Deluge-inal: One who produces a great deluge, or flood, of conversational utter-ances.

Disasterized: To cause or become a disaster.

DIY: Do It Yourself

Dopamine: The chemical deficiency that causes Parkinson's disease.

Fangster: A critter that possesses fangs.

Gloatation device: Mannerisms pertaining to gloating.

Goes-on-ta: The lid of a container.

Goes-in-ta: The container itself.

Gomer-style: A stereotypical habit of a shop towel

hanging out of a back pocket similar to Goober and Gomer Pyle from the Andy Griffith show.

Glub: A man's style of measuring liquids. When pouring something rapidly out of a gallon jug in makes a "glubbing" sound, hence the name.

Hobby-shopping: Working in the shop or garage as a hobby, not a business.

Honey-do: A project given to a man by his wife, "Honey, would you do this for me?" This is similar to a granny-do, a project at his mother-in-law's, and a sonny-do, something requested by his mother.

Insultation: The act of insulting some poor and hapless soul.

Insulteer: One who, or that which, insults with the skill and prowess of a musketeer. Which begs the question: Why did the three mus-keteers use swords instead of muskets?

Iowegians: People from Iowa.

Lucid, Lucidity: Clearheaded, rational, an interval of sanity.

Nagivator: A navigator, but the spoonerized version is more fun given the nagging nature of navigators.

Napper: One who spents unscheduled time in an unconsious state commonly referred to as sleep.

Novacaine brain: A brain numbed much the same way in which Novacaine numbs the flesh.

Myoclonic: Having to do with myoclonus.

Myoclonus: A neurologic jerk.

Oughta-do: A project that a man ought to do. Something that needs to be done soon, usually proclaimed such by the man when faced with a honey-do project.

Paradoxicity: A paradox.

Parkie: A person with Parkinson's

NPF/SD: National Parkinson Foundation South Dakota chapter.

PD: Parkinson's Disease.

Pretzelizing: The diabolical act of twisting one's words to mean something else than the intention of the one talking.

Procrasinator's Guild:

A ficticious organization of people who love to put things off. I made it up, so if it truly exists I don't know of it. And I haven't gotten around to researching it either.

Problematized: To make into a problem.

PWP: Person With Parkinson's.

Ridiculosity: Ridiculousness.

Schnozola: Nose.

Seniorized: Turned into a senior citizen.

Sniffer: Nose.

Sometimer's: A play on the term "Alzheimer's," meaning that a memory "sometimes" works and "some-times" doesn't.

Smurf: A blue cartoon character.

Snoozified: Rendered into an unconsious state commonly referred to as sleep.

Spoonerism: An unintentional interchange of sounds, usually initial sounds, in two or more words (Ex.: "a well-boiled icicle" for "a well-oiled bicycle") named after Rev. W. A. *Spooner* (1844-1930), of New College, Oxford, who was famous for these.

Stupidaline: An imaginary hormone that causes one to do stupid things.

Tandemness: Pedaling in tandem, or unison.

Use-ta-wasser: Someone who "used to" do some-thing or he/she "was" somebody.

Wackbards: A spoonerized version of "back-wards".

Wala-tada: A word of exclamation a magician might say at the moment of surprise, similar to the usage of shazaam.

Whifferama: A hypothetical contest where contestants identify smells.

Woulda thunk it: Slang for "would have thought so".

Yawnimals: Ficticious critters that cause fatigue, but are never themselves fatigued.

Yorkie-do: A hairstyle for Yorkshire Terriers.

Zoomster: One filled with boundless energy "zooming" hither and yon.

About the Author

The author resides in Sioux Falls, South Dakota, with his wife, Katie, and their Yorkshire Terrier, T-Bone Dickens. He is an ordained Baptist pastor and holds a Bachelor of Arts Degree in Theology. He served as pastor of a Baptist church in North Idaho for ten years, and currently serves in his local Baptist church. He also spends much of his time writing in various genres. He has had articles published in a variety of publications. He, also, serves on the board of the South Dakota chapter of the National Parkinson's Foundation, and writes a column called "Wanderings through My Ponderings" for the chapter's newsletter.

Website: www.KevinTBoekhoff.wordpress.com

Facebook: Kevin T Boekhoff, author

Email: ktbpub1@gmail.com

www.ingramcontent.com/pod-product-compliance
Lightning Source LLC
Chambersburg PA
CBHW070657290526
45790CB00001B/351